The Obama Kennedy Nation

The Obama Kennedy Nation

Can We Afford to Let the US Government Takes Over our Healthcare?

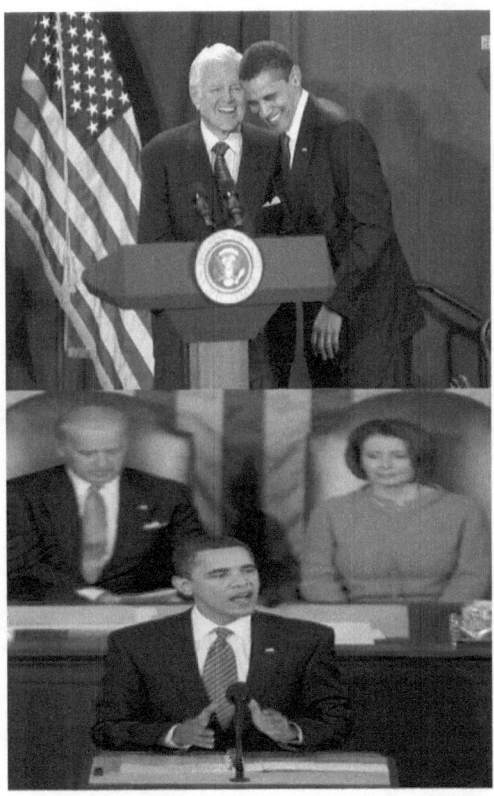

Medicine: the Science of God

Dr.'s 10 Commandments for Disease Free & Healthy Life

The American Health Care system

Can we Afford to Let the U.S. Government Takes Over our Health?

They Are Just not That Into the Health Care Reform

Top 15 Killers of Americans

The Best Investments

Immigration: a Healthcare, Economic, & National Security Issue

Things we Thought you Should Know

P.,P. Charly,

M.D. & M.H.A/Gerontology (*Candidate)

To order additional copies of this book, contact:
Xlibris Corporation
1-888-795-4274
www.Xlibris.com
Orders@Xlibris.com
68547

Contents

Dedication

This book is dedicated to my brother Jean, whose lost of the brain tumor battle did not influence his legacy and his commitment to my education and that of many individuals.

Acknowledgements

I thank God for my 73-y ear-old father, whose lifelong victorious battle over asthma does not prevent him from being the best hardworking father someone can ever have; his courageous support to my mother has proven to be the quality of the best husband, father, and friend to all of us. I also thank my siblings, relatives, and friends for their devoted supports and prayers on my behalf, from my poor teenage to my academically enriched medical and administrative studies.

Preface

In the Past 200 years, The United States of America has proved to defy the capacity of human to fully understand the almighty power of science and the Creator of the human race. From our mysterious independence to our first strip to the moon, Americans have grown to obtain the capacity of the leader of the world. As a nation who stands for freedom, liberty, and the pursuit of happiness, our leadership in proclaiming freedom and human rights has been, though its flaws, a success story. All over the globe, the name America had resonated power, freedom, and the land of opportunity.

Despite our ability to bring the torch of freedom, peace, and love to the human race, we have sometimes neglected our own children, while serving the most needed aboard. Love requires self-denial, and that is exactly what we do. However, charity starts with self, and this is proven in many natural laws of physics and aeronautics. "In case of Oxygen needs, during the flight, everyone should put their own mask in order to better help others" is the most common statement we receive from any flight crew, when we are ready to take off on an airplane. Therefore, as we are providing help to the needy aboard, we also need to provide ourselves the most useful survival kits of health care, immigration document, and educational formation about the subjects of which we are planning to get involved.

It is unacceptable to invest the most amount of our economy than any industrial country on health care, while struggling to provide care to every American. It is unacceptable to see that third-world countries we do provide financial supports, can provide better health care, immigration, and education to their people than our government do to the American people. We can do better than that! As an M.D. & M.H.A/Gerontology student, whose undergraduate in biology was full of extra-curricular activities, and work experiences in finance, real estate, and community services as radio health reporter, I have combined my life experiences with my personal dreams to write this book as a road map for the better America that President Lincoln, Washington, and the Kennedys fought for, in the unity of all states for a stronger nation.

Chapter 1

MEDICINE: THE SCIENCE OF GOD

The First Thoracic Surgery Ever Done.

During the first thoracic surgery ever performed, God put Adam to sleep and made Eve from Adam's ribs. That was the first thoracic surgery ever done, even before sin and the father of all evil were introduced to this planet. From history to anatomy, from physiology to pathology, we can see the God of creation is all over the molecular components of human existence. Considering the fact that pharmacology, in its flaws in harming too many people, one would ask two questions:

1) Is medicine really from God?
2) Does God really create the universe?

For the sake of argument, let's get rid of the 2nd question because it is so easy to answer. The easy and simple answer is: "yes, because God says so." "No Doc, you must be kidding," one might say. This answer can be given to the 1st grader, whose father might train him/her not to challenge what older folks have said or believed. However, if you were raised in family like mine where asking questions and questioning facts and beliefs were part of our daily hobbies, you will not take the above answer for a credible and sound answer without reasoning. Now,

It's time to *remyelinate our *neurons by digging in the mind for answers! "Doc, didn't you say that this question is the easiest?" you might say. Well! Can you remember the last time your Doctor told you something that was easy to understand? Very seldom, right? Okay, let's get to the simple facts then! Could this chapter exist if there was not a writer? Could this book be published if there was not a printing house? Could this bookshelf exist if there wasn't someone to build it? To keep it simple, let's just say: NO. No, that can't be! I guess we just hit the nail on the head. A chapter has to have writer; a book has to have a publisher and a bookshelf a builder. But this planet wasn't built by an architect? I think you might need to practice this answer for the Apprentice, because if you take a look at the NYC Trump Tower and say the same about Trump's marvelous building, he will look at you and say: "you are fired"

Unlike most other Doctors who just give you the treatment plan and procedures and are gone within 18 minutes before you can think of a question to ask them, since I am also an *MHA/GER student specializing in elderly care, I would assume that your amyaloid protein is acting up and cannot keep up with the *NYC speed. Let's compare this book to a BPL (Brooklyn Public Library) cart, and the earth to be a Boeing 747. A cart can be used and understood by anyone because it was made in China, where they contently pay employees $0.80/hr without benefits. On the other hand, Boeing 747 that FedEx uses to send this book overnight to you is proudly made in Detroit, Michigan, where the best and the finest hardworking Americans earn $8/hr. If the cart can be made in China and operated by the laziest driver, do you think that Boeing 747 is too complex to be made by the Americans, and is it fair to try to attack the Boeing makers? Oh, ok, I thought you didn't agree with me that Boeing, though complex to fly, was made by the Americans!

Now, let's get back to the bottom line and forget about all those *lead on questions Doctors use to make you speak your mind in diagnosing your actual health condition. If you believe that the simple cart, that may even be full of lead to poison our kids, can be made by the Chinese cheap labor, and the complex Boeing 747 has to be made by the world finest workers in Michigan, what makes you believe that this planet is too complex to be made by God?

As a Biologist, I know you might ask me: "How about the big bang? W hat about it! Are you telling me that when a sound was heard, pressure and heat were released

---

*   Remyelinate = covering sheet of the nerve cells
*   Neurons= brain cells
*   MHA/GER: MHA = Master in Health Administration, GER = Gerontology, means elderly care
*   NYC speed = New York City fast way of living
*   lead on questions = open ended questions asked by clinicians

to hit a mass of which its particles formed the universe, along with the earth? All of these coordinated stars, sun, moon, and planets, came from the existence of a crash? I will need to have a lot of faith to believe in such accident. Maybe this would be done like the movie of which, from the pieces of the FedEx airplane crashed, The FedEx Executive built his little house at the deserted island. Then, you are going back to the previous discussion. Then, you are telling me that, from the pieces of the Boeing 747, the executive built his house; this implies that, from the art works of a designer, another designer built a less complex piece of art. That makes sense. Maybe the maker of the 1st art work is the designer of the 2nd too. Therefore, one can conclude that, from that vocal bell sound, pressure and heat designed by an architect were released, and "bang!!! The universe burst to existence. I think I can buy that because it sounds like creation to me! Oh, you didn't mean that! Do you mean that it happened by genetic mutation? I hope you are not going to tell me that humans are from mutated monkeys because a 3 year old will ask you: "Why are the Bronx Zoo monkeys have never mutated to become an awesome American Gangster?" I think this belief would require so much faith, that many billion years of biochemistry research at the *Iowa AGEP would be needed to try to explain this process of which, I would rather believe in the preventive system of an actual creation where the sound was the voice of God, and the actions were that of his mighty hands.

"Who is this guy who has come with such creation and why did he created humans that has become a *pathogen to the universe?" some of us might ask. Unlike most doctors who would take the easy way out by saying that they are only here for medical care, and that question is for your bishops to answer, since many fellows assume I was going to be a bishop when I grow up, let me act like a medical student who is also a bishop in trying to answer such theological question. According to God, the Universe architect himself, the earth was created as a "tool" to prove that his love is that is given to anyone, even if they choose not to follow his plan. This is the great controversy between good and evil where God's love has been proven so good that even his greatest servant has been allowed to rebel and lead others to do so without fear of immediate destruction. That is why the earth was created as the aseptic battle ground between good and evil, between the Son of light and that of darkness. It is needless to say that this planet completed the creation of God's universe.

Medicine is an electron particle that came from the light created by the sovereign architect. As the matter of fact, the architect is reported to be the 1st thoracic surgeon by putting Adam, the only creature of God's image, to sleep and took

---

*   *Iowa AGEP = Iowa Alliance for Graduate Education and the Professoriate, a Summer research program*
*   *Pathogen = an agent that causes infection and diseases*

his rib that was cultured, cloned, and genetically modified to make woman, the mother of all. This sounds like the architect is an M.D./Ph.D. or a medical scientist. It seems like science and wisdom started with and came from the architect of all. That is why science is a great step in knowing the God who 1st used science in his architectural laboratory. Science is of God, and will never contradict the words of God, despite the powerful tricks of the prince of darkness to make us believe we should avoid science, if we have faith in the Creator of science. Although darkness particles have overshadowed the interconnection between God and the scientific evidence of his power, faith in dark scientology is so unreliable we would rather embrace God's account of creation instead of ten billion years of research to disapprove it. Now I know you want to ask me "how can it be possible for God to create the universe with a few simple words?" I will also ask you how NASA could build the space shuttle, which has not to obey the law of gravity? It's all about science baby! God said and bang it happened! This is God's powerful voice of his "big bang creation theory."

Chapter 2

DOCTOR'S 10 COMMANDMENTS

FOR DISEASE FREE & HEALTHY LIFE

I.   Sleep, Rest, & Stress management

No matter what is your mood in reading this book, you and I can at least agree on one thing: sleep and rest are the MVP, the first, and the last step of our daily lives. That is why, the Creator himself, although does not essentially need rest and sleep, has rested on the 7th day after creating the earth on 6 days of oral and hard physical labor. One can argue that God didn't do much during that creation week, other than one thoracic surgery that produced a woman, the most beautiful of all creatures, and thus did not need any rest. This is apparently a good argument, and it might really be the case. Without asking you to read 5 surgery books about the surgical process of separating Siamese twins, I rely on my medical background to tell you that most doctors don't really do things because they really need to, but to simply teach patients, enlighten nurses, and explain to insurance providers what is at stake if such procedures are not followed. As the matter of fact, if you read the Torah, you might observe that it wasn't until the Exodus of the Jews from Pharaoh's slavery that heavenly workers were reported resting on the 7th day. This sabbatical rest is an MVP for both heaven and earth. Rest and sleep were set for us and should be part of our daily, weekly, monthly, and annual routines.

No matter what is our lifestyle, the 6 to 8 hours of sleep per day is not debatable, if we want to live healthy. If you want to be healthy, start implementing changes in your rest and sleeping habits and, before you finish readying this book this month, you will see that health improvement. Continue to live happy and confident, but start working smarter on a timely-managed agenda, instead of working harder, you will see the difference. We might also need to put an end in having pride in calling ourselves "Blue Color Hard Working American" and start thinking about how we can manage our time to think how we can timely and efficiently use our technology to make things happen at a faster rate while putting fewer hours. In order to have a healthy life, we need to reverse the *pathological way of living to its initial physiological characteristics by providing enough daily and weekly rest and sleep to ourselves. We might also need to add some state-of-the-art vacation to our annual budget because we are going nowhere with hardworking that produce more stress than happiness. The purpose of life is happiness, and it is useless to gain all if happiness is lost in the crowd of business. If we want to claim back the American happiness, and the good health it induces, we need to slow down and start living. Although, inspiration is only 1%, while hardworking requires 99% hardworking, without thoughtful planning, hardworking cannot guaranty success. It is with good rest and sleep that we can make thoughtful plans. Stop listening to those of us who are New Yorkers and want to make you believe that the fast subway is the way to go. We need to ignore the late night shows, restaurant, and awaken. If we continue moving at such *oncogenic speed, we will not have time to think and act properly because our neuromuscular activities need rest in order to plan and make best decisions of life. By the way, did I tell you that stress is the # 1 cause of all diseases by shutting down the immune system and promoting sickness? No wonder why people who sleep better, get more rest, and live a stress free life are happier, healthier, and live longer. That's why! Have you ever believe that the world cannot survive for a few days without you? Book your next out-of-town vacation package and you will see that this planet will do well without your few days of input, as long as you live healthy enough to get back to your job. That is why you cannot afford not to have a vacation. The following are some few things that might improve your vacation quality and thus improve your health, work performance, personal relationship, and your critical thinking:

- Let coworkers, family, and friends know that you are away for vacation in order to avoid "emergency need calls," which could be taken care by others if you are absent.

---

*   *Pathological = related to disease development*
*   *Oncogenic = genes that cause cancer*

- Have "away on vacation" voicemail so that people won't expect your call back.
- Have automated "away on vacation" replied email so that people won't assume that their message have reached you.
- Turn off your Blackberry smart phone and prove to the electronic world that your vacation have been able to keep you a couple hours away from the electronic world, that can function without your input.
- Avoid internet, computer, TV, Cable News, and smart phone use while having quality time of relaxation and rest.
- Enjoy the exotic food by the beach instead of looking for the KFC or Burger King.
- Create more intimate and romantic moment with your life partner by visiting parks, zoos, museums, and sporting events.
- Share your vacation experiences with others, so that they can plan going with you next year instead of planning how to screw up your vacation time.

Do you think that you need to work two jobs in order to afford such vacation leisure? Not at all! As the matter of fact, if you need to work two jobs in order to make ends meet and have a vacation, you are already living above your means. You might need to budget your finance and reprioritize your agenda so that relaxation time can be part of it, instead of paying for the room you don't even have time to sleep on, because you are too busy working to pay for that expensive room. Relocation might also be needed so that you won't have to work two jobs to pay for the mortgage and SUV that you don't even have time to drive.

Talking about vacation, it is sad to observe that America is the only industrialized country that does not value vacation enough to establish laws that require annual paid vacation. Maybe lawmakers are too busy working for re-election, so that they forget to plan about vacation for America and thus destroying our health and working styles.

II. Water

Why don't we jump over the primary stress manager and diseases killer? Water is obviously known as the basis of life, but we have taken far for granted its healing power in such a way that dehydration has become the # 1 cause GI diseases in America. 70% of our body weight is water because the human cell and extracellular fluid count for about 70% water. Not bones, not fats, not protein, not sugar, but water is the major body component. I think you have already seen the picture! Even if we get everything else the body needs to survive, without that

7/10 that is water, we are not even close to the passing of any standard test with a 3/10 score. If we want to keep each of the trillion cells of our body satisfied, happy and healthy, we've got to give each of them that 70%, they are longing for! The question now is: how much water should we drink a day? Although it is not medically proving, we have been told that average of 8 glasses/day; the simple answer is true. Is it really true for everybody? Absolutely not! The simple reason is that this amount is based on the average weight of a 70 kg man with average lifestyles. For instance, if you tell Kobe that 8 glasses of water a day is enough for him, he will look at you and say like: "are you planning to make me crash and drop dead during the 3rd quarter so that the US Olympic Team and the L.A. Lakers would not see another championship?" on the other hand, if you try to make my 40 kg, 19 yr old cousin to drink 8 glasses of water a day while watching 6 TV Shows in a row, she will ask you if you are trying to make her spend more time in the restroom instead of watching her favorite shows. What I am trying to say is that we should drink just enough water not to ever feel thirsty because the spinocerebelar track send the "thirst" message to the brain when the endothelial cells have long been digging for water. This is because of the following factors about water in the body:

- Water cleans the immune system
- Water controls blood pressure
- Water controls digestion
- Controls the Genitourinary function
- Helps prevent infection
- Promotes body flexibility
- Controls fat absorption and mobility
- Controls sodium channel of glucose transport

III. Diet

What the heck is diet anyways? Unlike the prerogative term of diet in which people think of losing vs. gaining weight through anorexia vs. hyperphagia, diet simply means the way we eat. This term is synonymous to the word nutrition. Therefore a nutritionist is a dietitian. What is the best diet in nutrition? The following pyramid says it all in term of recommended daily value.

---

*   *Anorexia = starvation*
*   *Hyperphagia = eating too much*

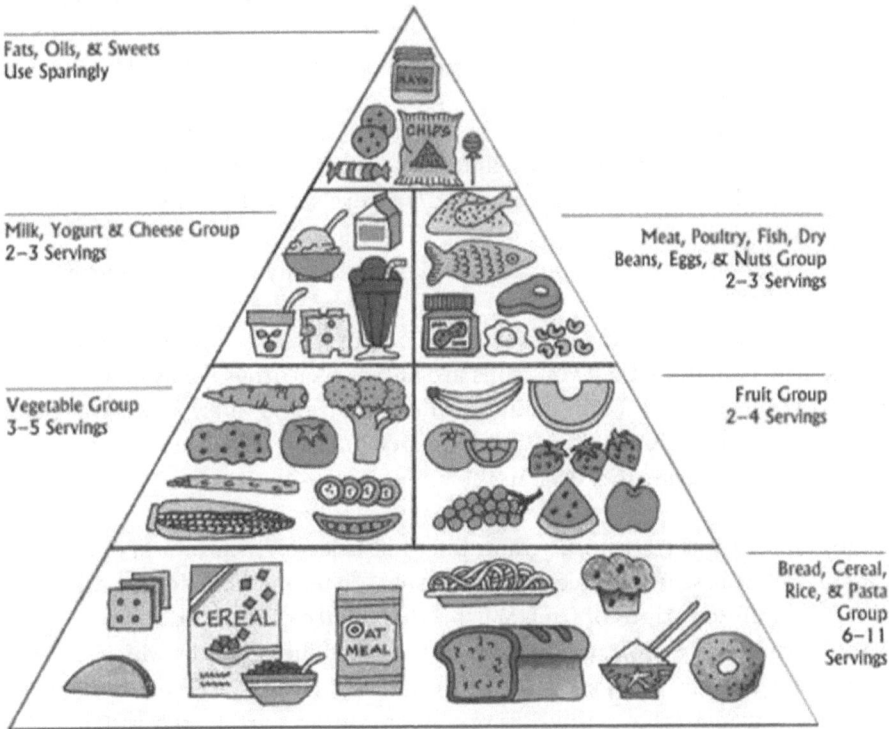

Fats, Oils, & Sweets
Use Sparingly

Milk, Yogurt & Cheese Group
2–3 Servings

Meat, Poultry, Fish, Dry
Beans, Eggs, & Nuts Group
2–3 Servings

Vegetable Group
3–5 Servings

Fruit Group
2–4 Servings

Bread, Cereal,
Rice, & Pasta
Group
6–11
Servings

Since, we, Americans, eat three times of the daily value eaten by other nations, I will not talk about the 2000 calories a day that most people embrace. Do you know that our tooth structures prove that meat should not even be part of our diet? I will keep it simple with the reality of portion in this matter of priority. Let's start with a few slogans!

- Eat one apple a day and keep your heart healthy enough to stay away from future cardiologist like me.
- If life drives you nuts put some nuts in your diet to clear your mind.
- Stop giving excuses in order to continue eating French fries, the worst fast food on earth, but made with potatoes that is the best food every existed.
- Instead of killing animals and eat them while letting them eat the good vegetables, agree to coexist with animals instead of playing survival of the fetus with meat diet.

---

*   *Food Pyramid*

- Even if you would put ten teaspoons of sugar in one glass of ice tea, you need to consider why your are still drinking soda pop that contains no real calories other than ten teaspoons of refined sugar that destroys your health.
- Stop the Dunkin' Donuts breakfast and late night dinner, and initiate the healthy breakfast and light food in cereal nightly dinner.
- Small frequent meals and daily exercise is the only road to lose weight.
- Diet pills only help starvation and dehydration instead of losing weight.

"What is the science behind these slogans?" might you ask. Apple is the prototype of the fruits family. If I tell you fruits are anti-cancer drugs, you will ask me for pages of biochemistry? I don't mind the details anyway. Fruits contain the major antioxidants, vitamins and cofactors needed for the immune system and all biochemical pathways that exist in the body.

Digestion of fruits starts in the mouth and lasts less than two hours in the GI. Therefore the best meal to take at night should not be one from the late drive-thru but from different kinds of fruit. What is the science of fruit metabolism? From early morning to 8 P.M., the body is in the catabolic phase by which all food consumed during the day are broken down to provide *ATP energy needed for daily activities. That is why, it is very important to start the day with a happy breakfast, just like we fill up our car tank before hitting the highway for a long distance trip. During the metabolic process, fat and protein are broken down into ATP so that the liver machine can distribute energy and oxygen to the brain, heart and kidney, the most important engines of the human body. What happens if we do not have a good morning breakfast and afternoon meal ? The liver call upon coal miners (hepatocytes liver cells) and middle eastern reserves (adipose cells) to provide some new energy sources through the *gluconeogensis process that will leave the body with free fatty acid, ketoacidosis, and cholesterol to stress our red and white blood cells, just like processed oil leaves us with green house gases and cold miners' disease. The only way to reverse this negative effect, is to have morning and afternoon meals rich in fruits, nuts, and vegetables because the brain is the engine that consumes ATP and oxygen as fast as they GM hummers and the NASA Boeings. Since glucose is the primary source of ATP and oxygen, fruits and vegetables are the primary sources of glucose, we can deduce why fruits and veggies should be our major diet. Here is another important factor that is not usually discussed. Except a few essential amino acids that we need in our

---

*   ATP = Adenosine TriPhosphate, the major energy used by the human body
*   Gluconeogenesis = glucose production from other sources

daily meals, almost all complex carbohydrates, fats, and proteins can be made by the liver machine as long as glucose, vitamin, and minerals from fruits and vegetables are fed to the liver factory.

Do you now see why people who eat fruit and vegetables have more energy, think smarter and better control there body weight? Just in case you might have not yet seen the light, here is another old school illustration. If you are told to buy some clean V-Shell Power from Chevron for your kerosene lamp for the cheaper price, and pay Ford to put that oil into there SUV Explorer before you can transfer this oil to your lamp for a few more dollars, you will scream and ask Washington D.C. for an bailout!!! But this is what we have done by asking the Midwest to provide us some pork and beefsteak after giving them the good grains and greens, and eat the animals' product as "good energy source". Is that the smartest idea to obtain energy from energy riched foods, or would it be wiser and cheaper to eat the grains and greens directly from the source without having to get the third party or the unreliable D.C. lawmakers to get involved? This is what I mean by that illustration. Fruits, nuts, grains, and greens are all the liver needs to make and breakdown all the energy needed for any healthy individually. Does this ring any bell about the young Prime Minister Daniel who won the healthy diet contest by eating only nuts, grains, and greens, while others were killing their arteries' and endothelial cells with animal products? I love Wisconsin, but the "eat cheese or die" slogan should have been "avoid cheese and meat to avoid disease and live". How about the myth "meat needs meat" or "flesh nourish flesh?" This is Fred Claus, who has been making us believe he has a brother called Santa Claus, who has met God on Christmas season to make good sell. There is no such medical or nutritional proof about meat. I wish the animal activists would know that truth, so they could be on the side Thanksgiving turkeys crying for a liberator. Let's look at one example. Vitamin B_{12} is usually said to be "found in animal products only." With the trillion dollar meat industry on the defense, though bigger the car industry, I would challenge the meat industry to give me one medical reason to continue to driving to them for B_{12} whereas GI normal *flora bacteria, nuts, grains, yeast and fish can each provide me one mail that is good for eighteen months. Oh yeah! One B_{12} meal can be conserved by the liver for more than a year because the body needs so little of it, and since it is a heat resistant fat soluble there is no need to crave a lot of it for normal nucleotide (DNA & RNA) synthesis. If you do not trust me enough to go meat free to be healthy, you can play it safe by taking some B_{12} supplement, Total cereal, and yeast components every once in a while. This will save you more time, money, and the stress required to prepare a meat diet. Also, when you feel like having

---

*   GI normal flora = bacteria that normally live in the Gastrointestinal track.

some M&M, do you think you want some sweet? No, you are actually craving for fat, which is found in the chocolate. IHOP has become the international house of obese people in feeding America fat and sugar. Do you know that America die on doughnuts that causes obesity and diabetes, though Dr. Jason have lost his job for telling the truth? Maybe he was fired because cops love doughnut; maybe making money by Dunkin' Donuts and the refined sugar business is more valuable to the American economy than the American health. Will I jeopardize my future in the medical field for helping the American people to find their way to good health too? I hope fat cops and public official will also get fired just as the Cleveland Clinic stop hiring obese people. However, I believe that we need to fight obesity instead of fighting obese people who need our support and cooperation to lose weight and resume a health body mass index.

IV. Exercise

Exercise is the key to good health. When we excise, we create a balance between the mind, the soul, and the body. Do you wonder why the cheerleaders and the basketball stars are the smartest, the kindest, and the strongest people of almost all communities? The secret is exercise. Just the smoothies taste better when we better blend it, exercise create a biochemical harmony with every neuronal, cardiac, *hepatic, and renal cells of the body. Remember that these 4 organs are the MVP of the northern to southern and the eastern to the western all starts of the human body. Starting from the *sarcomeres, exercise stimulates calcium ATPase enzymatic activities in providing energy for each muscle. When muscles contract, they mobilize the adipocyte to break down fat into energy because each fat molecule would give 9 ATP and many more oxygen molecules. Do you already see why some exercise gives us a lot more energy? Do you already see why people who exercise would burn their fat storage and thus lose fat and weight? Do you already see why doctors tell patients with high blood pressure, arteriosclerosis, heart diseases, and diabetes to exercise? That is the science behind the above medical orders. How about we start with normal healthy people and follow up toward acute to chronic pathological condition? With a 45 minutes of exercise, a healthy individual make and conserve energy for about 22 hours, such that each minute of exercise produces about 30 minutes of strength and energy. That is simple math to me, though medical students and math are not the best political rivals! What is a healthy individual anyway? Medically speaking, people are considered to be health when their Body *Mass Index (BMI) are between 19 and 25 without pathological condition. Someone is underweight, when

---

*   *hepatic = liver cells*
*   *Sarcomeres = skeletal muscle cells used in contraction*
*   *BMI = Weight in kilogram/height in meters squared, (Kg/m^2)*

their BMI is under 19, whereas being overweight requires the BMI to be above 25. As mentioned earlier, healthy individuals break down all food sources into glucose that would later be broken down into ATP energy. When we exercise, our body uses the water we drink, the oxygen gas we breathe, and combine them with glucose to produce energy during the first 20 minutes of exercise. Since protein and ketone are concentrated and locked into the liver reserve for the moments of starvation, fat are the most bioavailable molecules our body obtains at its disposition during the next 15 minutes of exercise. Therefore, about 35 minutes after we start exercising, fats are broken down very fast in the catabolic process of exercise. You might remember that each molecule of fat can produce 9 molecules of ATP and oxygen. Can you imagine how many ATP and oxygen energy is produced during that last 10 minutes of exercise, if a billion fat molecules are broken during each second of physical activities? Thy is why we, health care professionals, usually advise people to exercise 30 to 45 minutes on a range of 3 to 6 days a week.

Have you seen another connection between fat and exercise? The more we exercise, the more fat we brake down for energy production, and the more glucose and protein we make and reserve for the next day. As we brake down fat, we will automatically lose size and weight, while building lean muscles because muscles are mostly made of proteins. Protein looks good in the classroom, the workplace, the field, and the bed. This is where the confidence, self-esteem, and real beauty start. If we burn and mobilize fat during physical activities, cholesterol related to diseases such as obesity, diabetes type II, atherosclerosis, and cardiovascular diseases will fly away from from our body and dive to the swine. Hopefully, none of us will go after that meal in the Iowa pork market because swine flu is on the watch! Did you also know that when cholesterol is mobilized, it is converted into steroid and sex hormones during the anabolic process? This anabolic process starts at 8 PM under the neurotransmitters called serotonin and melatonin. Do you wonder why, when we go to sleep, we wake up with a sex drive? Do you wonder why Kobe, Gov. Pitzer, and Gov. Sanford got themselves into trouble with their wives after waking up next to other woman after a good time in the gym? I think this exercise regimen is more affordable than Viagra and fertility pills to me!

Do you think that I forgot to tell you about the power of exercise on our brain? As the matter of fact, since the brain is the MVP of the body, I think we should know a lot about it. However, it's best to leave the brain section to the part dealing with mental health, because telling you that the neurotransmitter endorphin is activated by exercise in order to think, act, and behave, would be a simple give away. That is why we would ratter let you relax you neuron in looking forward to stretch it out in the study of neuromuscular diseases.

V.   Sunlight

Sunlight is the major energy activator of the human body. Have you seen how much energy and power Sarah Palin brought to D.C. after she breathes the some southwestern sunlight from McCain? I am just kidding! I am not going to get you into the politics of solar and wind system although we all enjoy the "cash for Clunkers CARS program." When we expose our body to one hour of sunlight, we have activated enough energy for a whole week. How is this energy activation occurred anyways? Vitamin D, for instance, is the major permissive switch that works with thyroid and parathyroid hormones to turn on energy sources for molecular activities of every cell in the body; however, even with the best diet and exercise, vitamin D still requires sunlight to be activated, so that it can stimulate every biochemical pathways within the human organs. Do you see what would happen if we lose that sunlight activation? All circuit will be busy like a Sprint or AT&T iphone, even when we own one the Apple monopoly of all food. I don't mean to be too conservative, but we will use that "old school" illustration to better understand the importance of sunlight in our lives. Have you ever heard your grandma talks about how good her clothes smells and how long they lasted when she used to dry them on morning sunlight? Maybe you are like me and were not lucky enough to know or meet your grand parents to share their lives of wisdom with you. Maybe older parents might annoy you so much with their inconvenient true of their wisdom, that you have exiled them to a nursing home. Whatever they case may be, doesn't really matter for this conversation.

What I am trying to say is that the sunlight is the best purifier of our external and internal body organs. Most anti-oxidants of the immune system depend on the sunlight to better protect us against diseases and keep our skin melanin clean, our keratinic vision, and our mind and heart healthy. However, we should remember that too much of a good thing can be harmful; just like too much oxygen on ventilation machine can be harmful to respiration, we should avoid too much A-wave sunlight that ages our skin, and B-wave that can burn our skin. That is why, if especially we have fair and light skin, we should limit our daily sunlight exposure or apply sunscreen to black the harmful waves of the sun. We should note that #15 sunscreen is enough to cover up to 95% of the sun waves. It is not cost effective and medically needed to buy a # 16 or more sunscreen in order to have an extra 1% that can also be blocked by our skin immune system, while paying a few dollars more on an expensive sunscreen. This is marketing strategies to make us believe that we can bell-ourselves-out of skin cancer by spending a lot of money in pharmaceutical products to protect our skin. As the matter of fact, some of those cosmetic products only increase our risks of skin and other diseases.

VI. The Power of Alcohol

I know you think that I am going to start with the same myth that is destroying the American society by saying "alcohol is good for our heart." This is just a lie that we have been trying to explain for thousands of years. People try to prove their point by taking stands along quotes from holy books without letting you know those ancient writers were talking during a time when grape juice was purely made, without adding any synthetic alcohol that wasn't, by the way, invented until the 17th century. Although I have a French background, I cannot keep that secret from you! Louis Pasteur and Jenner were the first to study bacteria and yeast in there natural way of making alcohol in the cellular process called anaerobic glycolysis of ethanol fermentation. You might recall from previous sections that glycolysis is performed by bacteria normal flora of the GI track. Do I even need to tell you more in order to see that? If we drink enough grape and citrus juice, the normal flora will loyally continue the process for our heart, while we are busy making big bucks in wall street or main street. Another truth about the delicious French wine is that we would need to drink 200 gallons of wine, 100 gallons of beer, or 560 shuts of whisky in one day in order to to provide enough *Resveratrol for a healthy heart while alcohol would destroy our normal mucosal flora. Not to say that we would die right away with such daily alcohol, if liver cirrhosis and pancreatic and kidney cancer would not kill us by then, the Dallas cowboys cops would have to chase after us in I-30, until they find out who allowed us to drive with such alcohol level. Maybe, one thing we have not been told is that the French people are too handsome and arrogant for us to stop drinking their wine, or we might not have access to the arch gate of the Midwest if we let Budweiser and Miller Light go out of business. Budweiser is no longer an American company anyways!

Although, I know you are going to say that I am here as another doctor to scare you, do you know that alcohol drinking is the major cause of accident? Do you know that alcohol is the #1 cause of cancer and liver failure. If you are the Apple CEO who can get on the top of the list for liver transplant, you might not need to be worried about finding a new liver from the NJ mayors and rabbi. Do you know that alcohol drinking causes more long-term harm to your heart and mind than any other ingested materials? I know you are now calling me the messenger of bad news, without realizing that the *FDA and *NIH are those who release such data whereas they continue to license the alcohol drinking industry.

---

*   *Resveratrol = cardiogenic chemical that promote health and immunity*

*   *FDA = Food and Drug Administration*

*   *NIH = National Institutes of Health*

Just in case you didn't know, it's never been about our health, it's always all about making money. If it brings money to someone's bank account, they will let it fly by until it takes over, just like Michael Phelps' use of pot create the national debate of legalizing marijuana, instead of punishing him for acting stupidly and violating federal laws. Do we need to start a debate about legalizing dog fights or should we wait until Michael Vick brings a football Olympic MVP to America? How about legalizing the use of surgical anesthesia drugs to treat insomnia and facilitate Michael Jackson death? Maybe this could stimulate Michael Jordan return to the NBA or eventually the White House after a disastrous divorce.

Enough of the sarcastics, though, it is the best heart medicine, so that we can get back to the alcohol drinking issue. If the government knows all those negative effects of alcohol, since we are talking about health care reform, shouldn't we start eliminating the major causes of diseases and accidental death, instead of such status quo of disease care system? Although he is getting as old as John McCain and cannot pursue one campaign without cancelling the the other, my dad once said: "instead of hiring doctors and nurses to mop the floor after the mess made by alcohol, drugs, and unhealthy lifestyles and diets, we should use doctors and nurses on what the are best at—promote disease prevention and help treating the unpreventable diseases."

Since I stepped into Joyeux-Depart Kindergarten over 25 yrs ago, I have observed that students who drink alcohol are not good learners just as teachers who drink are not good instructors. I have also come to observe that drivers who drink alcohol are as abusive to the road as parents are to their children when drinking alcohol. Needless to tell you that Washington D.C. lawmakers who drink are not going to make final calls in favor the American people who elect them just like Professor Gates was not able to listen to the 911 call of his people after participating on the "Muller Light Beer Summit" in Obama's White House with the MA Policeman who was typically under the influence of alcohol while arresting the Harvard professor. HWB*(Home-owner-While Black) is not typical to DWB*(Driving-While-Black), unless the police officer is under the influence of alcohol in the arrest of the Harvard Scholar, while he was opening the door of his own house, that wasn't in foreclosure jam by the collapsed Countrywide Mortgage Company. Do you see the underline issue with alcohol? Its only good purpose in life is to put us in trouble, get us arrested, buy us, and sell us at a deadly price. Just go to CNN, Fox, or utube to listen to Joe the Plumber, who has no plumbing license or Joe the Vice-President, who has no cerebellum, and you will see that alcohol has no place in a healthy society where people need to think before doing and saying things that makes sense in a healthy society.

VII. Smoking

Health and smoking should not even think about going out on a date because these guys have no character compatibility in a healthy society. When we look at the biological damages caused by nicotine, tar, and other dangerous gases produced by smoked substances, you might ask this question: "How in the world smoking is still not prohibited in all levels of the American society?" A friend of mine would tell me smoking is a human right. Maybe it is a right to kill self, and others! Is it because the Collapsing economy of Carolina depends on the tobacco industry to survive? Is it because we don't have the gut to chase the drug cartels in our Mexican border? While chronic bronchitis, asthma, and cancer are destroying American health, the government prefers to tax the tobacco companies, while the Cable Media, with the shameful help of Michael Phelps, is promoting the legalization of cocaine, marijuana, and heroine used at the expense of our health care system.

Did you know that alcohol and tobacco companies pay our elected lawmakers more money than their taxable salary? Do you also know that taxing tobacco does nothing but enriching the industry? While we are busy adding 1% tax on tobacco, this industry is busy adding 3% sell price, and 30% cancer cases and 60% more cardiovascular cases, which will all combine to destroy our family's health and economy.

VIII.   Family

"First things first," is the new slogan in promoting family value in America. When we hear family, we usually jump over the thoughts of responsibilities. On a medical point of view, family is more than just a few responsibilities. If it would have been about responsibilities only, when our children move on their own, family mission would have been over until grand children would be born and start asking to spend the weekend with grandma or go playing with grandpa. Medicine and clinical psychology have proved that people who are family-oriented do not only decrease their risks of diseases, but also promote their health improvement when affected by any physical or mental illness.

One of most important factors of family is the communication between family members. I am not talking about the email, instance message, voicemail, letter, and text messages. These are channels that count for only about 15% of communication. More than 85% of communication is non-verbal. Real communication requires body language and facial expressions, which help people to see and feel the confidence and fear during a conversation. The real communication happens at the dinner table, the living room and the bed, where actions talk and the mind visualizes the outcomes. To improve communication, family members should spend more time together because the more we do together is the better. If a picture is worth a thousand words, an action is worth a thousand pictures because your action says more than you can even think of!

What is the biomedical influence of family over the human body? In the previous sections, we explained how stress is the primary factor of sickness. Let's now take the time to differentiate positive and negative stressors in the context of family value. Positive stressors are any physical and mental factors that activate our brain neurotransmitters. When these transmitters are activated, they send signals to all peripheral nerves and muscles to call crossbridges for the work being done. Anatomically speaking, nerves and muscles are co-dependent in such a way that, if a nerve is not active, it will slowly die and cause the muscle it enervates to *atrophy and die. The reverse is also true; when a muscle is inactivated or damaged, the nerve that supplies electrical impulse to the muscle will eventually die. When we have a family, it is very unlikely not to have a family member who has a physical or mental work for us. These works maybe to take care of the grandparents, take the kids to school, take the dog for a walk, prepare a meal for dad, search on the internet for mom's latest home improvement, and so forth. As you can see, each of those activities has something to do with one group of muscles or part of the brain.

Those stressors are made to stimulate our neuronal cortex in such a way that the frontal lobe that is in charge of personality can fully be used, when the smart 3-year-old starts asking all kinds of questions about the IPod, or when the 80 year old grandma has attitudes for not dressing up according to her Vietnam War Era. This is where the parietal lobe will be reminded of which president was in power by a simple look by the occipital lobe to the picture of grandpa's room, while his temporal lobe is busy listening to the NPR news updates. Wouldn't family stressors be part of our lives, those of us who are still single or busy working for Uncle Sam, would not have the adequate challenges to the mind and the body. This would create muscle atrophy and nerve degeneration as self-destruction because challenges are made to make us stronger and smarter. How about the since of belonging that we feel and loss when going on a business trip without family? It is not until we are locked alone at the Marriott resorts during a vacation or business trip out of town that we fully realize how much family really worth. Family is a major factor in helping us think positively and set standards for success. Remember to set high standards because we will never reach certain standards unless we set it ourselves. If our marks are set high, we might require

---

*   *Atrophy = shrinkage and death of a muscle*

several trials and error in overcoming difficult steps that might be painful along the way. In the process, we need to be humble enough to ask others for supports and sacrifice other profits, which would hinder us from reaching a higher point of goals. Destiny is a matter of personal choice, instead of an unbroken wall set by nature against human in order to make us feel helpless in changing any situation. Impossible is only found in the mind set; we are capable of changing any situation, no matter the opposing circumstances. Like doing physical exercise, the courage to go forward and the strength to persist are found in overcoming each challenge of life. The more we succeed or try to succeed, the more strength we will have to keep trying until we reach the highest mark. That is why we need to be persistent and have the determination to follow the right direction toward success, love, and achievement of our goal, even when the odds are against us. Family and friends are the most valuable tools to have, when we positively use their ability to make a difference in our lives.

Those who are divorced or separated can quickly grasp the destructive power of being away from our own family, no matter how difficult it was to be around them. I know your mind is wide open to ask me: "how about those negative families where the Phoenix hot sun is cooler than their heat and pressure?" it is sometimes true that some families have brought negativities to our lives. On the following, I know you may not agree with me but we have also agreed to disagree. Negative stressors are made to make us stronger too.

Yes, negative people and circumstances only slow us down more than helping us; but, we sometimes need to slow down in order to see the 10% negative while we focus on the 90% positive. "But the only thing they see is that 10% negative in our lives," you might say. Let's have the audacity to hope that those specific people are not among those you chose to be your soul mate! For, any other family member will be, one day, in a different path of life, where you positivity would never have to collide with their negativity on a D.C. Town Hall meeting. For that temporary time they spend with you as parents, siblings, friends, or a community church member, you can recall that microscopic picture that was only seen by those people with their skillful negativity and talent of negativism. "Are you telling me negativity and pessimism are skills and talented gifts?" some of us might ask. Those gifts might be given to the blue dog democrats and old dog republicans. Are you agreeing with me simply because I turned on the political switch, or does this illustration remind you of that family member who skillfully advised you not to marry that lovely Joe or beautiful Jenny who turned into a WMD or a diva to Bush and Cheney while their daughters are respectively

---

smoking Michael Phelps crack, and professed to be an homosexual while carrying a lovely child. Is it because of those negative behaviors among family members that push President Clinton, and Governor Pitzer and Sanford to destroy their family, or is it a consequence of not valuing family? Maybe, only a diplomat like Hillary can explain to them that if we value family, we can become the senator of the greatest state, even if we are not resident of the state that make us famous again to the level of presidency and the share of power with the greatest mother in the White House.

Family oriented people do not only have 74% more chances to succeed in life, but those supports provide the right neuronal effects that the neuromuscular junction our heart and kidney need to operate for a healthy balance. This biochemical interaction is proven, when we visit a family members at the hospital bed or the encouragement given to a love one before a surgical operation. Do you wonder why elderly who move to nursing home have a less healthy life, more infections, and die faster? This is the power of family. America needs to wake up to build family value, instead of building wall street that is going to be destroyed again by Madoff and Stanford financial scams.

IX. Forgiveness

Love forgives and forgiveness brings happiness as the happy heart is the best medicine. Like President Mandela and Secretary Hillary Clinton, forgiveness can give you power over people, over enemy, and over yourselves. Power over self is what the soul needs the most, to regenerate the nerves of our mind, on our thoughts process, and body on our lifestyles. If we want to be happy, we need to start forgive ourselves like Kobe Bryant, Michael Vick, and Governor Sanford and stop quitting on ourselves like Governor Pitzer over a night stand with a call girl, or Governor Palin, over a year touchdown with the wrestling media attacking her family, and conservative values. Like Senator Ensign, we need to take step on forgive ourselves in adultery attempts and acts.

When we don't forgive ourselves, there is a since of guilt that keeps following us throughout life. This guilt will eventually attack our confidence, and later our self-esteem and purpose of life. This self-destruction will not only create loneliness and suicidal thoughts, but also stereotypical, discriminatory, and hatred behaviors in the hallucinated mind just like someone who is under the influence of drugs and alcohol. Forgiveness, on the other hand, is the best therapy of the soul; it gives you a sense that you have the connection with a higher power for a higher purpose in setting the mind to look at the forgiven person as a lower being that we control, even at their most critical behaviors. When we forgive, endorphin and serotonin transmit the message of relief from the mind to the cardiovascular system, which eventually decrease our blood pressure and promote vasodilatation by the penetration of oxygen to the cells.

Do you now know why we take a deep breath when are stressed or upset? Since we already understand the stress mechanism and its correlation to blood pressure as the primary factor of cardiac health, we can also postulate that forgiveness is a divine prescription to the soul in providing good health to the mind and body. If you wonder why people enjoy being around you, increase your volume of forgiveness and you will see the amplitude of call back you will receive from good old people who were waiting on you to make the 1st step to resume the broken bonds. If you wonder how self-forgiveness can affect your health, start making a list of the many things you used to blame yourself on, you will see how the mind will reset the forgiveness pathway of the upper motor neuron for a renewed lifestyle initiating new objectives and purpose of life. The power of forgiveness can be illustrated using the metaphor of an infidel ex-husband who receives a "get well soon" balloon after a DUI car accident. This man maybe so hopeful that "things" maybe forgiven and work again that he can't wait to get well very soon, in order to reach out back to his ex-wife, who has potentially forgiven his adultery. His neuromuscular vesicles will fire so many acetylcholine that the damaged *diaphragm and *myocardium, will get well so soon that she would wonder whether he did not pretend to have damaged organs to seek forgiveness from a *carcinogenic and *teratogenic behaviors.

X. Trusting God

When our Ford Explorer or F-150 are giving mechanical trouble, though tune-up, oil change, and supreme car care, we read the owner's manual or contact the "Michigan Big-three" factory to make sure our car is not among any "recall." When Aspirin regimen is not efficient enough or intoxicates our liver, we contact the Fleming Rx Company and the Aspirin distributors for in-depth analysis of the drug *Pharmacodynamics. When, despite our strict application of preventive health and healthy lifestyles, sickness threatens our lives, we need to request help from the manufacturer and Creator of mind and body. This is where faith plays critical roles in our health and disease improvement. Those of us, who are already faith based individuals, know that disease started in the Garden of Eden when our parents were manipulated to disobey the law of love of their Creator.

---

*   *diaphragm = thoracic muscle of respiration*
*   *myocardium = heart muscle*
*   *carcinogenic = cancer causing*
*   *teratogenic = harmful to fetus and new born*
*   *Pharmacodynamics = the drug does to the body*

Just as putting diesel on a gasoline engine, ingesting unhealthy ingredient in the body would deteriorate our body. Since the sin strand was injected to the genes of our forefathers, we were doomed to be sick and die of the cancerous oncogenes forever, unless the Creator would provide the chemotherapy and surgical radiation of his Son as a healing treatment to our humanity. When we are sick, suffering, and dying, this is not a punishment by the God who created us, but it is simply a reminder that we need his medical intervention for our soul, mind, and body. Sickness and death are the ultimate consequences of our inherited lifestyles and behaviors. Collagen is the most common triple stranded protein of our body. When we have needs, the Father, Son, and Spirit are, like 3 strands making collagen, standing there awaiting us to call upon their supports. The blood of the Son is transferred on our heart, so that DNA evidence on rescue and investigation would not be of ours. Simply claim his support and call it a day, he will get you through.

The 1st step toward good health is a healthy lifestyle, along with behaviors as proposed by the user's manual of our maker. When our weakness and self-exposed temptation deceive us and prevent us from following the user's manual, our maker is always ready to redeem us and "recall" our heart, mind, body, and soul for maintenance. This renewal and maintenance might require recalling the engine of our heart and replacing our plasma with a new blood. This healing method is available to all of us just like GM is ready to recall any troubled engine and gives us a new one. All that is needed is to filling out the request from and ready to pay the maintenance fees through the change of lifestyles. Doctors, health care professionals, religious leaders, and political leaders play all a role in the renewal process by helping us following medical treatments, moral principles, and community based activities for a healthy living.

You may wonder what political leaders have to do with your spiritual, physical, and mental well-being. Just visit the TN River Park of Chattanooga, the Miami VA Hospital, and the Brooklyn Down State Medical School to see how good government policy can improve health, while training the brightest to for the highest mental abilities. This is where we will see the relevance of a good health care system in America. Just as observing God's 10 commandments is not sufficient to take you to heaven, following the above 10 principles for a healthy living is not perfect in itself. That is why we need a good health care system in America.

Chapter 3

THE AMERICAN HEALTH CARE SYSTEM

What is a health care system? The world system is biologically explained when we take many chemical compounds to make organelles that are organized to form living cells, which combine to form the organ systems of the human body. Like the human body and parts of a car, every administrative setting has many components that combine to form a system. Therefore, medical schools, doctors, nurses, drug companies, health insurance providers, government agency, and health institutions combined to form the health care system.

There are several kinds of health care systems in the western world. The most common ones are socialized medicine, single payer system, government funded system, private medicine, and multi-sponsored competitive medicine. In America, we have the multi-sponsored competitive health care system where the government sponsors a certain group of people whereas employed and self-employed individuals respectively buy their health care insurance through employer-sponsored plans and personal premium. Despite its drawback in several medical aspects, the American health care system is the most solicited by people from all over the world. Why is that citizens from countries like Canada and Western Europe, which are said to have better health care system, prefer to obtain medical care in America? The first answer is that we have the best medical technology in the planet. The second reason is that we have a health care system well-suited and fitted to the capitalistic economic system of the 3G world. Because of that competition, health insurance, pharmaceutical, and medical institutions have to improve their customer services to compete at a national standard, on the basis of cost effective medical care. In other words, America is the only industrialized country where you can get medical care at the speed of a fast-food restaurant. Just as fish sandwich lovers like me have the choice of Berger King, White Castle, or Mc Donald to buy a meal depending on how much we want to spend at a certain time and location, in America, health care is served as fast as the hot patty in Times Square. Therefore, people of descent academic, and more importantly, of descent financial background can obtain the best health care services in the planet. Just like buying car insurance, people who are buying health insurance premium can make a side-by-side comparison on the quality, reliability, and the price of the health care coverage and services.

Can you see why this speedy service attracts all nations to come to America for medical care? The reasons are simple. If we have sufficient fund, we can get all the coverage and treatment we want in America. That is why Canadians and Europeans come to America because their systems, unlike America, is on the 1st comes 1st served basis. Can you imagine having the best coverage or the most money and have to wait in the line to be served at your zip code after Joe, the alcoholic is served? Doesn't this kind of service ring a bell to you? How about the U.S. Post Office, *DMV, and Public Transportation? Now, you see where I am going! Luckily, we don't have such waiting in the American health care system. Is it because it is not government run system that we don't have such waiting? Not at all! We simply have a system that is set for success, no matter who is in charge; however, there is a problem here. If the smart from overseas, the rich from Wall Street, the famous from Hollywood, and the educated from Cambridge can go across the medical spectrum for a better health care coverage and care, how about the talented sons and daughters of Joe, the alcoholic who live in the project? "This ain't my problem! They have a congressman who gets paid to serve their district problem," some of you might say. Well, well, well! Is the H1N1 infection staying within their zip code, bus route, and local mall? Is the corona virus infection staying within the Summer Redbox of their neighborhood? I guess not! As long as Joe's children go to the magnet school you children attend, they share the shameful burden of being uninsured with your household.

Maybe it sounds unfair to you to pay the consequence with someone else, but infection doesn't care about who commits the action. Maybe another metaphor would better help us grasp my point in explaining what is at stake in not fixing the health care system. In defending the legacy of his father, President Bush destroyed the legacy of Collin Powell in sending our troop to hunt for oil tanks

---

*   *DMV = Department of Motor Vehicle*

in Iraq's anthrax dost. Now, secretary Gates has proudly taken our troop back home, along with all kinds of germs from the Persian Gulf. Do you think having a good health care system for our veterans is an issue that should concern all Americans? I guess we should say thank you to the lawmakers who were inspired for the Veteran Affairs and their hospitals. I guess the veterans' health is not the only one that affects all of us. If so, how come the veterans have the best health care, whereas their brothers and cousins, who take care of their children and looking after their household while they are serving, cannot have a share of that health care opportunity? It is because we want the veterans to be too busy taking care of their relative so that they won't run for office? Maybe, we just want to increase their post-traumatic stress disorders in struggling supports to their sick relatives. Like the VA, Medicare, Medicaid, and the children health insurance that cover over 30% of the population, we need some kinds of health care program for the other 40 millions of uninsured American.

Medicare is a federal health insurance program for people 65 and over, certain people with disabilities, or patient with end—stage-renal disease. Medicare does only cover a large part of medical expensive. Medicaid, on the other hand, is a government health insurance that helps low-income people in the United States to pay their medical bills. Despite the fact that the Federal government creates guidelines for the program, every state has its own rules. The rules vary from age to health states, from immigration status to financial background.

We can all observe the fact that that the VA, Medicare, Medicaid, the children health insurance, and the federal employee health insurance are all government run programs, and count for over 32 % of the population. When we add that 32 % to the 60% of privately covered Americans, we can proudly say that over 92% of the American people have some kinds of health care coverage.

Among the above groups, the VA is reported to have the best and the most flexible medical services, after the ironically called "the Cadillac plans." The success of the VA system is partly due to the fact the VA system have its own hospital facilities. The Cadillac plan that is sold to the richest Americans, count for about 5% of the American population. The Cadillac plan is of good quality simply because those rich and famous people are able to pay for the flexible, but expensive health plans. Although this plan is over 46 times more expensive than the average premium, it is so reliable that every medical provider across the globe accepts this insurance plan. The congressional plan, provided to the executive, legislative, and the lawmakers, is as efficient as that of the Cadillac plan. It is common sense to see why lawmakers vote for the best health care plan for themselves. The only problem is that this plan doesn't last if a lawmaker is not re-elected.

Although costly and partly inefficient, Medicare, Medicaid, and the children health insurance are adequate medical coverage and are partly flexible. Funded by the government, these groups of people can select their own doctor as primary care physician, medical facility, and pharmaceutical services, as long as those factors abide to states and federal health policies and medical standards.

Therefore, we can stipulate that over 35% of the American people have an efficient medical coverage that is the best one in the standards of the new world. The other 57% from the total covered people have a limited premium that cannot be evaluated, until customers have need for medical care. These kinds of coverage vary by many factors, which include age, ethic group, state of residence, profession, and health conditions. Health condition is the ultimate driving force in shopping a premium for this population. Most people of this group assume that they can purchase the health insurance they want, until the insurance agents would ask them a few health-related questions and reply: "mom, I hate to tell you that but your family health condition and lifestyles prevent us from providing you any coverage at this moment; we advise you to contact another provider." Can you imagine how stressful would it be not to be able to find a Geico, Progressive, or an eSurance plan to cover your old Buick because you just replace the transmission of one of your cars? Car insurance companies don't give progressive those 15 minutes of second thoughts to give you some kinds of plan for your Buick, because the Geico would offer a 15 minutes quote to save you 15 % on your car insurance. This is so easy; a caveman can do it on care insurance!

You might also wonder how in the would the health care reform would likely happen when the White House is losing points for being on the right side of the issue? Do you wonder how health reform would ever happen, after the death of Senator Kennedy, the filibuster proof vote and the most out spoken advocate for reform, have gone and left us alone in this battle? Anyways, can the White House afford to be on the wrong side? Unlike Hillary Clinton, who was not an elected official when she was trying to reform the health care system 17 years ago, this government was elected for that mission, among others. Shouldn't we repeat that to the deafs of D.C. whose temporal lobes is not quick in hearing: "this government was elected to primarily fix the American health care system. Let's explain this opinioned statement. When Hillary, who has a special training in health law, which she 1st used in the State of Arkansas, she assumed that the D.C. bulls were as cool the Midwest cowboys. Therefore, the 1st Lady thought that her charm and beauty would impress the Tom Delay and Tom Ridge machines, whose perfect loyalty to the supporting insurance lobbyist won't slow down for the Clinton political machine. While Hillary was, behind closed doors, busy trying to negotiate a health care reform, Monika was gaining sentimental ground in the White House as the poll numbers against President Clinton forced him to drop the "Hillary Care," that Bill Frist and Newt Gengrich ate alive. In compensating for the Clinton health care massacre, *NAFTA was given as a *placebo to manage the disease of the American economy that has come back with health complication. However, this placebo made America feel so good that the carcinogenic destruction of our economy by NAFTA could not be seen until the Carl Rove ravage destroyed our immunity with two wars, after 9/11 and Katrina took our confidence away from us to send it to China and other cheap labor countries. President Bush spent so much time studying speeches prepared by Rove and Laura that he had no time looking at the Wall Street greedy behaviors. Sleepless Rumsfeld put President Bush to sleep with some holy scriptures in making him believe that he was destroying the American values and that of the world in the name of God. I know that the radical morons of Jerusalem and that of the Arabic World believe that, but when was the last time God ever relied on the weak human race to fight for him? The God of love and peace is not in the business of war, famine, destruction, and pesticides. That is why we need to be in the side of God to fix the pesticide of the broken health care system that is killing over 8% of the American people.

I know you might be saying: "we are doing pretty good in covering 92% and the other 8% can go to the emergency room, if they need help." Don't be in the side of the retarded Rush Limbaugh by promoting destruction to the economy of the individual states. As a medical student, let's explain this economy issue on a physician point of view. Because of the settings of the American health care system, anyone who does not have health insurance and needs immediate care can obtain it at the expense of that hospital. If that patient is not qualified for Medicaid, such as self-employed and under-employed people, the hospital is required to carry that bill, and thus charges other patients higher cost in order to cover that medical bill. We can therefore see how everyone in America would obtain care for a higher cost because of the emergency care for the uninsured. If that same uninsured E.R. patient is qualified for Medicaid, the state of residence would be forced to cover that care that would not have to reach critical care level, if the patient was covered for primary and out-patient care. That is why Medicaid is reported to be the biggest burden every state has to carry. Because of the cost of avoidable Medicaid-qualified E.R. care, states like Florida and New York have to cut research on diseases like cancer and HIV/AIDS in order to balance their emergency health care budget. In more critical economic conditions like this recession, some educational programs, such as that of charter school and student meals have been cut in balancing state budget in treating preventable diseases.

---

*   *NAFTA = The North American Free Trade Agreement*
*   *Placebo = Effect produced by inert tablets*

Another issue of the American health care system is that too many test and diagnosis are being performed in taking care of patients. Most of the tests are simply done because doctors and hospitals are playing it safe in making sure medical lawsuit and malpractice claims do not follow their philanthropic and humanitarian efforts. Although a "simple sorry" or 5 more minutes of conversation with a patients could have reduced those lawsuits, doctors order several test for the same diagnostic purpose in insuring the 1/1000 relative error of the medical technology could be avoided. If health care professional use the power of communication, they can explain those error analysis to patients and reduce the cost of running several different tests for a disease diagnosis.

Malpractice Claims

In talking about malpractice claims, we should also mention that health insurance companies increase our premium in order to cover the malpractice claims. Since malpractice claims count for ¼ of the cost of the American health care, if we manage to reduce the number of health claims, we can drastically reduce the cost of health coverage in America. An important fact that we should note is that about 90% of all medical error claims have been denied. Isn't there an underlying problem here? If most malpractice claims are denied, lawyers and judges are not out there against doctors because, apparently, the medical system has been the winner of it all, except 10 % of all cases. Why is that? The answer is that most patients, who claim malpractice on medical errors suits, simply do so because they feel mistreated. We all know that feelings do not always tell the true reality. If patients lost 90% of malpractice claims, the problem is not the patients who file the claim or the lack of performance and knowledge of the lawyers and judges, nor lack of training of the doctors. The primary problem is a matter of information, education, and communication among health care professionals, patients, pharmaceutical companies, and insurance providers.

Information is the basis of knowledge. When doctors and hospitals spend adequate time to inform patients about the management of their disease, they will understand that doctors are rather trained to improve instead of declining the health of the patients. Let's take the car metaphor again. When we go to a mechanic shop about our care transmission, a good communication with the technician will help us realize whether fixing, buying a used one, or order a new transmission. Whatever is our choice, we all can deduce the time, cost, and quality of the transmission after the mechanical repair. Just as all good technicians would explain the outcomes and guaranty of each repair choice, well-informed patients would already predict most medical outcomes even before they sign the informed-consent form provided by the medical facility.

Education is another aspect in both providing care and avoiding medical error claims. Patient rights, for instance, are information that most patients don't really understand until the day they make that phone call to the law office about their "mistreatment." In their willingness to help others while making a living, lawyers would bring the patient rights to the attention of their clients. Since most medical claims are about those rights, feeling of patients are mostly hurt by finding out that they were not educated about their rights while receiving medical care. Would patients receive adequate education about health care, many medical issues, prescription drug errors, disease complication, and malpractice claims would be avoided.

Communication is power. Those of us who have large families, have been involved in community activities, or have been involved in team projects have experienced the influence of the powerful weapon of communication. The Japanese proverb says that "a kind word can warm a winter season." Even when people strongly disagree on issues, if there is communication, there can be compromised or simply "agree to disagree" without fighting in front of someone else, who did not witness or cannot even make educated decision about the actual issue. Without putting American finest lawyers on the defense, we all can arguably note that most lawyers and lawmakers don't have enough understanding of the complex health care system to make sound 3rd party decisions about conflicts of health care and the care quality definition between patients and doctors.

What I am trying to say is that doctors should help patients understand medical issues through informed and educated communication, so that trust can be built between patients and their doctors. Lack of trust produces fear and rebellion. This trust will improve the health care quality for our nation by decreasing medical errors, lawsuits, and disease complications that are mainly caused by lack of communication between patients, health care organization, and medical professionals.

Medical Errors

Medical error is a very sensitive topic because, although error is the domain of the human race, nobody can easily agree that they make mistake. People usually compensate by blaming their errors on the errors of somebody else. When it comes to health care, errors is truly a multi-stage issue where many people are actually involve. The biggest errors in health care come from the lack of communication. Instead of improving communication, technology has nowadays destroying it. Instead of one-on-one communication, where body language and facial expressions can tell the confidence and fear, people prefer the email, voice, and text messages to communicate. College Communication 101 has thought us that words count for only 15% of communication. If 85% of communication is non-verbal, how in the world would we expect to have excellent communication, while using only 15% of its accessories?

It is sad to say that medical errors cause more accidental and preventable death than any disease in America. The following are the most common medical complications caused by medication:

- Rx toxicity
- Rx to Rx interaction
- Rx allergy
- Rx poisoning
- Wrong diagnosis and prognosis
- Prescription Rx misunderstanding

As you can see, most of these errors are factors that are independent to doctors. We all can agree that a lawsuit against a doctor and hospital who remove the right breast or kidney, instead of the abnormal left kidney is a very fair case, but a Rx allergy blame should not be on the shoulder of the doctor. It is fair to cancel the practice license of a doctor who amputates the wrong leg, but should the Rx side affect be blamed on the doctor? The answer is absolutely no. Doctors don't make and approve drugs. Doctors simply apply FDA approved drugs using the guidelines of their facility and the National Institutes of Health (NIH). When therapeutic index of a drug is of a small range, it would not be theoretically précised to know if a specific ethnic group would experience toxicity. Allergy is another generally complex medical issue that doctors might not be able to predict and monitor, unless signs and symptoms are reported. This is where drug quality plays a critical role in providing good health care services.

Prescription Drug Incidence

Doctors prescribe drug but they cannot predict drug incidence that is only found on the data analysis of the pharmaceutical companies. Let's take the Real Estate metaphor for this section. When we need to buy a house, we contact a real estate advisor to better select a house. Since the realtors were not present during the building process of the house, they will only rely on secondary sources and local market data values to help us chose the best house. The accuracy of our housing choice is very limited due to the simple fact that real estate agents, who help us find the house, are not the primary sources or builders. This is also true in the health care system. Doctors rely on the FDA, *CDC, and pharmaceutical data to

---

*   *CDC = Center for Disease Control*

select the best medication to their patients. As often reported, if drug companies provide bias data to the FDA and CDC, doctors will typically not know all the facts about such bias until the prescribed drugs harm patient during a lapse of time.

The most unfortunate scenarios can be illustrated about drugs which cause harmful effects that do not present with quick signs and symptoms such as cancer, hypertension, and cardiovascular diseases. Because of the slow physical presentation of these diseases, doctors would typically not be able to monitor side effects induced by the drugs. Such effects are so common that the government would have to closely evaluate such drugs and eventually pull those drugs off the market if the pharmaceutical companies do not correct such common drug effects. How often such cases are true anyways? Maybe after the drug companies harm a couple million patients and make a few $ billion to pay the treatment or burials of the drug victims. This is where most American got killed by harmful drugs that are unintentionally or deliberately done by pharmaceutical companies across the board. Why is the government letting this happen so often? Might it be because the elected officials receive more money from drug companies than the sour taxable salaries?

Another incidental factor that harms patients is found in medical errors where doctors prescribe the wrong dose or the nurses follow the wrong medication procedure. With the use of information technology, the electronic system is already being adopted by many medical facilities in America to reduce medical errors. As the matter of fact, researches have proved that electronic prescription can decrease medical errors and their harmful effects by up to 30%. The problem is that electronic system is costly in both purchasing of computerized tools and the training for their usage. Is cost the most important factor or is health improvement more important?

We can arguably say that saving lives is the most important purpose of care, and it should be done at all cost. "Who is going to pay for it?" you might ask. Since doctors and health care professionals are making descent income while using their computers to bill patients, we should also agree that doctors should be required to use such electronic system for the improvement of health care, instead of improving the credit card billing method of profits. We, Health care professionals, are the best disciples when it comes to following standards. All Washington has to do is to make these good health laws, and we will follow the standard with either our own purchasing of such equipments or government funded programs through taxes collected by Uncle Sam.

Doctors are the best money savers when it comes to their own money and that of their patients. The American health care system would have been in better hands, if doctors, instead of insurance and drug companies, would manage our health care. The use of generic drugs is a good example. A generic drug is a drug that is created according to the exact *Amount of Rx for result of a previously created drug. During the preliminary studies of a drug, companies use many trials and error procedures to come up with a drug dose that works for most people whereas some people only need a fraction of such dose for therapeutic effects. Generic drugs have the exact number that is need for such therapeutic range, without that extra costly amount of drug that is present in the prototype brand medication. In addition to that, the first few costly stages of studying that drug invention are already done by the prototype drugs for the generic drugs. Therefore, generic drug designers can just put the exact tools equipment in chemical compound to make the drug without facing the hassles of trials and errors involved in the costly study of a drug. However the generic drugs work as good as the prototype brand. This is typical to buying all the parts from GM, in order to make your own car without running a Detroit factory expense which will eventually require a government bailout. The next time you stop at the Wal-Mart, take a look Tylenol and Nyquil that are both of the same acetaminophen percentage but the price varies. I'll bet you get the same treatment with a different price! "Why are doctors not prescribing generics only?" you might ask. The simple answer is that "money talks!" Since there is no agency other than your drug and insurance company, they manage to buy your health from each other, while the doctor gets a vacation package out of the deal. What I really mean is that brand drug companies cut a check to doctors each time they prescribe their drug, instead of the generics whose price is kind to the average person.

"Is a generic drug safe enough?" You might ask me. As a matter of fact, generic drugs, because of their low drug amount are reported to be safer for most people. That is why they are called over-the-counter drugs (OTC). OTC is a drug that can be safely taken by most people without any physician follow up on toxicity and side effects. Since medicine has never been perfect, there are rare cases where only the brand drug can be used; but such case are so insignificant on the average of the health improvement of the patient. This is where professional ethics is needed the most, so that your doctor can make the call on whether you should take the brand or the generic drug without the influence of a pharmaceutical or insurance company.

The Absolute Power of the Insurance Industry

The most powerful factor that influences healthcare in America is the insurance industry. Unlike many countries where care is the priority, the American healthcare system has been slowly becoming a money machine that takes the healthcare power off the hands of the patient and doctors. It is unfortunate that doctors no longer treat patients according to the medical trainings and ethics, but mostly according to the insurance policy that the patient potentially have. I say "potentially have" because not even lawmakers of our nation really know what their own healthcare covers, until they have medical needs. It is also sad to see how such lawmakers have the gut to defend and lobby for the mysterious insurance companies. Some of the self—imposed regulations in the health care providers are the following:

- if you change jobs you are no longer covered.
- If you lose your job you are not covered
- If you turn 18 get off parental insurance
- If you have pre-existing conditions, you cannot be covered
- If you do not meet the deductible, you will not be covered
- You need to contact us before seeing another doctor
- Before any medical procedure, talk to us before you set up care with your doctor
- If your doctor do not contact us before taking care of you, the bill is going to be on you
- Preventive medicine is up to us instead of you and your doctor
- If you get terminally sick, we may cancel your insurance policy
- If you get too old, we might cancel your policy

Therefore, after the insurance companies will select the above, what is really left in the population? You are covered as long you never get sick, you never grow up or older, or simply you never need healthcare. Let's see it this way: how will you feel if the GEICO reptile would tell you that you cannot get car insurance if your Chevy Malibu is getting too old or had an accident a few years ago. I guess none of us will ever get such car insurance notice because insurers know that the progressive jeep is waiting behind the GEICO reptile to jump in. Monopoly is what has been controlling the health insurance market in America. If there were at least a few options which cover the above conditions that count for about of 65% of America population, in order to stay in the competition, most companies will provide descent coverage to individual groups no matter of their health condition. By the way, how come the transportation department makes sure that every car in the street is insured and driven by a licensed driver and the health department allows such risk of letting these people circulating without medical coverage? Is our car health more important than our own health? How can we make sure that everyone around the corner is covered before H1N1 flu infection attacks us through uninsured people?

Can we also have a caveman in D.C. for health care reform? Here is the trillion $ bell-out question. Is your car more important to America than your health? Although buying cars keep Detroit factories alive, and driving to work keep the economy alive, I still assume we should have been given more health insurance options than car insurance. Buying a million new cars on the Cash for Clunker Program can save the country $1 billion a year if each car help save $3 a day on gas, I still believe that saving lives is more important than not sending $1 billion to the Middle East and decrease 1 billion less greenhouse gas to the environment, even for me, a Biologist. Although re-hire 1300 GM laid-off workers to re-open the Pontiac plant from the Cash for Clunker profit is good for a GM come back, I still believe that America should prioritized health care over financial care. What I am trying to say is that, just as every car in American road has insurance, no matter the model and the condition of the car, every American should be provided the opportunity to have some kinds of health coverage, independently to their pre-existing conditions. This is why health care reform in America is imminent, and we can no longer wait for Washington to decide for us on a political battle ground. We need to act now!

The potential problem is that if we don't act now, self-employed and under-employed Americans who cannot afford this status quo will start quitting on themselves and America. If we let the blue-color American quit on working hard by seeing that their hard working cannot provide health care to their families, they will stop working and rely on Medicaid and government welfare to survive. Are we ready to add another 50 million people to the government budget? Are we ready to pay 50% of our own income to take care of those uninsured hard working Americans? If we do not act now, this is what is going to happen because the middle class continues to work hard instead of asking for government bell-out like the greedy Wall Street Investors who collapse the economy. We need to remind the Obama government that they were chosen before the economy collapsed in order to reform health care, immigration, and diplomacy. If they are not ready to bring us the change we voted for, they need to help us find Nick Romney and the republicans to take over because they have the Congress, the Senate, the White House, and the Media. All they need now is step outside political interest that cannot re-elect them, if the American people select another leader.

The Patient Bill of Right

A Patient's Bill of Rights is a statement of the rights to which patients are entitled as recipients of medical care. Typically, a statement articulates the positive rights which doctors and hospitals ought to provide patients, thereby providing information, offering fair treatment, and granting them autonomy over medical decisions.

PATIENT BILL OF RIGHTS

1. **Information Disclosure.** *Consumers have the right to receive accurate, easily understood information and some require assistance in making informed health care decisions about their health plans, professionals, and facilities.*
2. **Choice of Providers and Plans.** *Consumers have the right to a choice of health care providers that is sufficient to ensure access to appropriate high-quality health care.*
3. **Access to Emergency Services.** *Consumers have the right to access emergency health care services when and where the need arises. Health plans should provide payment when a consumer presents to an emergency department with acute symptoms of sufficient severity—including severe pain—such that a "prudent layperson" could reasonably expect the absence of medical attention to result in placing that consumer's health in serious jeopardy, serious impairment to bodily functions, or serious dysfunction of any bodily organ or part.*
4. **Participation in Treatment Decisions.** *Consumers have the right and responsibility to fully participate in all decisions related to their health care. Consumers who are unable to fully participate in treatment decisions have the right to be represented by parents, guardians, family members, or other conservators.*
5. **Respect and Nondiscrimination.** *Consumers have the right to considerate, respectful care from all members of the health care system at all times and under all circumstances. An environment of mutual respect is essential to maintain a quality health care system.*
6. **Confidentiality of Health Information.** *Consumers have the right to communicate with health care providers in confidence and to have the confidentiality of their individually identifiable health care information protected. Consumers also have the right to review and copy their own medical records and request amendments to their records.*
7. **Complaints and Appeals.** *All consumers have the right to a fair and efficient process for resolving differences with their health plans, health care providers, and the institutions that serve them, including a rigorous system of internal review and an independent system of external review.*
8. **Consumer Responsibilities.** *In a health care system that protects consumers' rights, it is reasonable to expect and encourage consumers to assume reasonable responsibilities. Greater individual involvement by consumers in their care increases the likelihood of achieving the best outcomes and helps support a quality improvement, cost-conscious environment.*

Chapter 4

CAN WE AFFORD TO LET THE GOVERNMENT
TAKE OVER OUR HEALTH CARE?

Can we really afford to let the government take over our health care? This is the issue of national debate. However, the 1ˢᵗ question we need to ask ourselves is: "who is really in charge of our health care system right now?" is it on our own hands and that of our doctors, or the hands of the mysterious insurance and drug companies? I hope the previous sections of our discussion allow you to see that we and our doctors don't have the power over our own health, compare to the powerful and mysterious insurance and drug companies. To be in control of our health, we should have been able to choose insurance providers, instead of them choosing us as long as we don't have pre-existing conditions, risk factors, and unavoidable professional background. Controlling our own health care is not only about cost and medical care flexibility; it is also about human right. Our doctor appointments should not be on the hand of a third party like the insurance company or governmental agency. Such decision should be made by our doctors and us, according to our health needs, agenda, and lifestyles.

It is unfortunate that insurance companies have unsuccessfully controlled the health care for Americans. If their job would have been successful, we would not have this kind of discussion about the above failed health care issues in America. The trillion-dollar-question is: "can we really trust Washington D.C. bureaucrats to control our health care?" I wish Washington would have built that credibility of trust. Therefore what do we do now? Should we let healthcare roll like Chrysler, Wall Street, the banking, and the housing system until the healthcare system collapses in the hope of finding a 50 trillion dollar bailout from Washington? I guess President Obama will ask Rumsfeld for a Bible verse to pray for that to happen after his term in the White House. Since President Obama is more willing to lose political points now in opening this healthcare debate that cost Hillary the White House, It would be wise to take a chance with this. Since the pre-existing health condition issue killed Obama's mother, we can at least trust that he will eliminate that insurance issue before it kills his mother-in-law and million Americans mothers, who cannot be covered under the status quo because of pre existing conditions such as cancer, HIV, and diabetes. I guess Magic Johnson will be more than happy to share his Cadillac plan paid by Burger King with the American people. I know you care so much about insurance and drug companies who makes 400% profit this year while increasing our premiums by 200%, even though you are trying to make ends meet during this financial crisis. I would care much more than you do, if my medical Sallie Mae student loan and my uninsured neighbors were sponsored by any drug or insurance company. That's not cool to say, because these companies create thousands of jobs and should be fairly treated. That is better said now?

How can we have it both ways by having private companies and government sponsored insurance options? Wouldn't this draw the private companies out of business? Absolutely not! This is a manufactured fear tactic paid by the insurance industry who sponsored extremist right wing leaders like Rush Limbaugh, Sarah Palin, Glenn Peck, and many others who have been used scared tactics of WMD to invade Iraq. As a health care administration student, let me use some data to prove these people wrong before I become the Limbaugh to pick on TV and radio talk shows.

- The U.S. Postal Office does not draw UPS and FEDEX out of business but simply provides a more cost effective option for those who cannot afford a $ 25 fee to send a package across town via UPS and FEDEX.
- National public Radio (NPR) simply challenges Voice of America Radio to report competitive breaking news across the board.
- Public broadcasting Services (PBS) is just another local channel on the side of ABC and CBS.
- C-Spain is only reporting what CNN is competitively reporting on cable TV.
- The 24/7 NYC subway system is an alternative to any New Yorker who cannot afford a $20 taxi fare to ride from Times Square to Madison Square.
- The US Military Academy, although among the top 5 American colleges, does not affect the success the success of Princeton University in respectively giving the refined John McCain and Sonya Sotomayor to the American Public Service.

- Public High Schools, instead of limiting the performance of private academies, have both provided America the best 3 first ladies for the past 15 year history of the Western World.
- U.S. public medical schools, such as the University of Iowa, have provided an increasing standard by competing with private universities and training America's finest physicians.
- VA hospitals, though among our nation's best and most efficient medical institution, do not hinder John's Hopkins hospital to provide Siamese surgical separation.
- Community teaching hospitals like Down State Medical Center of Brooklyn does not affect the excellent medical training provided by the Brookdale University Hospital.
- The U.S. highways do not jeopardize Amtrak train interstate services in connecting the American coast.
- Medicare, Medicaid, VA, and the children's health programs have not put the private health insurance companies out of business, but closely work with AARP to better combine public option like Medicare with supplementary United Insurance plans in order to cover our senior citizens.

I guess the above examples are enough us to help us understand the underlying issue around the healthcare debate and the urgency of having a government funded option. Just as we see it in the Postal Office virus the UPS illustration, people who cannot afford the Magic Cadillac plan that is typical to the UPS price can smoke some Phelps weed, while in the post office line waiting for a $4.00 priority diagnosis of the Obama nation. If Blue Cross and Blue Shield insurance is that good in insuring all people, why aren't they confident to take that Princeton virus Naval Academy educational challenge on the healthcare level? I guess they will be required to improve services instead of increase cost, just as UPS and FedEx are being challenged by the US Postal Office on cost effective efficacy.

That is why we, the American people, should grab the debate from D.C. and bring it home so that the same republican politicians, who arrested us in Los Angeles for protesting the Iraq war, can get out and remembering that America voted for change. Those so called blue dog democrats should get out of the way before Chicago politics mash their career as Governor Blagojevich and Palin. Washington should also know that President Obama knows the game from food stamps request to "The Audacity of Hope" that brought change to the nation capital and the American prestige even at the Berlins wall in saying "Yes We Can." The President should also know that the polls are like the stock market that goes up and down, but the Iowa cornfield is the vote that really matters to the American people.

If we were ignored while protesting the chasing of the erratic Sadam Hussein regime, we might sometimes need to get arrested in order to sit down and listen to the elected leaders. We elect leaders so that they can make sound and wise judgment in our behalf, when we cannot foresee or are too busy to dissect the cable news and the internet to make informed decision. Having said that, the best way we can give our input is to listen and debate with the elected officials and challenge them to understand our doubt, so that they can analyze and compare options for a better America. If their decision does not respond to our needs, we can recall them home and replace them with new leaders. "This is easier to say than done" you might say to me. Let's look at this way! If the Republican president of the past 8 years would have the gut to put his republican congress at to work to at least initiate a debate on healthcare reform, President Obama will not have to embrace this heavy load. Why don't we ask the supporters of the status quo to draw back, so that the Obama and Clinton machine can finally find a way out to healthcare reform; thus, we can quickly fix our broken immigration system, before Lou Dobbs and George Lopez kill each other on the southern border about FEMA (Find Every Mexican Available) on Katrina clean up. The faster we fix immigration is the better because it is correlated to healthcare. When all Americans are insured, people will not have to go to ER for H1N1 vaccine or NSAID painkiller for arthritis. If immigration is fixed, we do not have to be worried about H1N1 illegally crossing our southern Mexican border.

Can the Government Manage Health Care?

Can the government Handle and manager our health care well? The quick answer is yes because researches prove that the VA medical system, that is a government-run program, has been one of the best healthcare services around the world. You might say that the military services are special cases but, like Medicare and Medicaid with implementing management, we have the potential and money to own the best healthcare system in the planet. Unlike the claim of many agencies, the problem of our healthcare is not money; America spends three times the money other industrialized countries spend on healthcare, whereas we rank 30th among the world class health care systems. The major problem of our healthcare system is the lack of management and regulations. This lack of management is within medical policies and standards, medical centers, drug companies, and insurance industry. Most drug companies spend most money in marketing their product than improving the major risk factors of the drugs. Quality and customer satisfaction are the best marketing strategies. However, drug companies favor money over health quality. Nowadays, insurance companies spend more money in bureaucracy that helps them find ways not to cover people than improving health coverage. Hospital and medical schools spend more time and looking for financial outcomes than using doctors and nurses for what they should be trained for: providing healthcare to America.

Politicians, on the other hand, care more about the health corporations, instead of looking after the American people and the small businesses which create 70% of the American workforce. If big industries count for only 30% of the job market, when will the government stop prioritizing the big Pfizer and other helpless guys needs over that of the majority? Even though individual families have followed the righteous pathway, if bigger health care entities are not at their best, we will never become the best in the health care services around the world. We have the best technology, education, and democratic systems that set the basic standard for success in all life issues, including health care. Let's step up to the plate and make all the changes so that those who are reluctant to lead will follow us in reaching the highest standards of health care set and dreamt by President Lincoln, President Washington, and Senator Kennedy. Let's give Senator Kennedy that gift he has been fighting for 30 years in dreaming to have health care for all American.

We can honestly agree that America needs a health care reform. Although honesty is the best policy, honesty is not enough when action to improve our honest mistakes does not follow. At least for the past few months, it is proven that we have an executive government that is willing to lead in changing Washington, D.C. through financial regulation, health care reform, education, housing reforms, and immigration. As the word executive sounds, the President can only put into action what lawmakers have decided. We need a congress and a senate that works. There is no excuse to accept this from lawmakers to pale around issues, such as health care, and immigration that affects every American family. The greatest need America has is a need of leaders. Leaders who want to change Washington, from being a city of political bully to a city of leadership for implementing short term and long term changes for a better America. America wants leaders who cannot be bought or sold by any institution. American needs truthful and honest leaders who are not fear of calling immoral behavior by its right name. We need leaders who are true to duty as needle to the pole and ready to stand for the right things, even if they are threatened to lose their job, fame, credibility, and their lives, just as our troops have done for our freedom.

Washington has too many lawmakers who are being bought and sold by pharmaceutical, insurance, and financial companies. America has too many leaders who dishonestly lie about executive policies that don't fit their agenda, or that of the companies which compensate their vote. We have too many leaders who prioritize re-election over the needs of our great nation. If Tom Ridge and Powell can confess to the American people, this proves that the hole of lie is not deep. There will be a day that true will prevail about each action we commit to manipulate the American people to protest against their chosen leaders. Let's see some of the lies being advertized against the President to reform health care.

Euthanasia by the Government?

Is the government-run public option plan going to promote euthanasia? The quick answer is: "absolutely not!" this is a scare tactic used in the 1990s by the pharmaceutical companies and the drugs industry to call the Hillary plan, "socialized medicine." If you ask, Lindsey Graham, the smartest and most honest southern politician in Capitol Hill, he will tell you this so called "death panels" that kills elderly are the same bitter movement agencies sponsored by special interest groups financed by drugs and insurance companies. As we all can see, these movements have created such distrust in the Obama presidency that the successful stimulus plan, "Cash for Clunkers" is demonized by saying that the government use such data to spy on the American people like German Nazi. These kinds of conspiracy theories have been promoting "black euthanasia" in many southern states, without perception of the illusion and inaccuracy of their message because the president is arguably black. The black euthanasia theory did not work to stop the election for change. The elderly euthanasia theory will not work to stop health care reform in America. We have hope that political leaders will learn from the McCain/Palin lesion. Until one month after her nomination for Vice-President, Sarah Palin was America's favorite governor, with a 90% approval rate until those right wing extremists used her and the McCain campaign for their own agenda, which destroys McCain and Palin political power, legacy, and their voice for the American people.

To make our euthanasia topic easy to understand, let's remind America that the Berlin Wall has fell many years ago. There is no way in the Western world politicians can survive in lying and manipulating people to promote euthanasia. Manipulation doesn't work because, when people see the light, their strong will turn against the manipulator. This so called euthanasia bill that President Obama has been blamed for, is a "Do not resuscitate" informed consent that was proposed by a southern congressman from GA. To set the medical ground on the issue, many states around the countries have already provided such health proxy and procedure, when patients and their family agree not to use some medical apparatus, such as tube feeding, AED defibrillator, etc. if this already in place medical treatment procedure was proposed by a republican lawmaker and supported by everyone, how do the republicans managed to allow special interest groups used them to drop this ball on Obama's White House regarding his support for this program? How come such bill that is less than 2% of the health care reform has taken over the overall health care debate? How come the President is letting this happen? Maybe he is too cool to be upset! If you think so, you need to ask Biden about the steel in Obama spines, or ask Hillary about her answer to the African student on Bill Clinton foreign Policy.

As mentioned earlier, this simple politic of fear is that of special agenda groups that are destroying American values for their financial and socio-spiritual interests typical to the Taliban in destroying the Middle East. Taliban, Al Qaeda, and the extremists are destroying the Muslim world for their own political and socio-spiritual gains. In any angle we look at it, this is flat wrong and will never please the God these groups claim to serve. These groups are religious nuts. The God of our faith is looking for spiritual fruits, instead of religious nuts. Spiritual fruits include the love for sharing ours with others. Love is sharing of our money, confidence, honesty, and health care insurance to the less unfortunate, instead of trying to destroy anyone who is willing to take political risks to help people in providing NAFTA in the 90s, invading Iraq in post 9/11, or in stimulating the economy this year. Don't you know that when presidents fail, America fails? If the Limbaugh movements are to fail America, we should not stand in his side. By the way, since our senior citizens are already covered by the government-run Medicare system, they should have been the least population to be worried about medical reformed because Medicare is already under strenuous reform.

College-age and the low-income are the major classes of uninsured that need healthcare reform the most, because they cannot be covered with the status quo. It goes back to the Iowa cornfield vote: "the college-age and the lower middle class were the two main ethnic groups who voted for change in America because they have been the victims of it all whether in fighting for freedom, working in our factory, or studying in our science labs. We should advice Washington to reform healthcare, immigration, education, military, and continue to improve our economy. If they don't do so, we have Mayor Giuliani and Governor Romney waiting in the line to rescue America, if this government is slowing down because of Washington scare tactics.

How About the Doctors?

You might ask: what is the role of doctors in healthcare reform? Because of the complication of the healthcare system, patients, government and community leaders have tendency to see doctors as part of the problem instead of the solution. As a medical student, I can honestly tell you that the actual healthcare has many factors that would not give doctors much option than following the failed medical pathway. Before we go any further, it is very critical to say that our failed system is still potentially among the best healthcare system in the world as long as new management is put in place. As mention earlier we have the best technology and provide the best medical training and we spend the most money in healthcare. The only drawback in our healthcare system is the lack of management, coupled with greedy corporations which use the healthcare system as a money machine, unlike other nations systems which obtain money as a bi-product of an excellent healthcare services. Since medical professionals, such as doctor and nurses, are the only people patient literally see, we have the tendency to blame our doctors for failed policies induced by federal and private agencies.

Starting from the beginning, medical schools need financial and academic settings where training doctors and nurses are prioritized over financial and soci-political factors. For instance, to become a cardiologist a doctor would have to spend over 200,000 dollars during the course of their twelve years of medical training. Let's us see it from this angle. If you allow a doctor to get out of an cardiologist fellowship training with $200,000 dollar student loan, that would equate 600,000 dollars in the issue of 10 years in high interest loan repayment. We can honestly agree that doctors will also have to drive toward where money belong, instead of better healthcare during the cost of that 10 year loan repayment cycle. We also know that any habit that last ten years has automatically becomes a lifestyle. On the other hand, if doctors and nurses would have obtained academic and financial support for medical training, as it is in most countries around the world, they would have a different financial mindset. If we sponsor their education we could also impose standardized healthcare that are not money driven but health oriented. In other words, insurance and pharmaceutical companies would no longer be the doctor checkbooks and the student loan consolidators.

In addition to studying, the failed insurance and medical systems have almost hindered doctors' ability to provide good healthcare without being concerned about medical lawsuit and malpractice insurance. When doctors have to spend ¼ of the annual paycheck to pay for malpractice and private practice insurance, it becomes very unlikely to expect doctors to follow health oriented decision instead of financial outcomes. As long as doctors have to face anxiety that would be too stressful, they would not be able to make the best medical call for the American people. That is why reform is need in the way that doctors will provide care to America. If third world countries, whose healthcare are funded by American agencies, can provide cost effective adequate healthcare to their people, the American people can and must reform healthcare system for an healthier America.

How About the People?

What role we, the American people can play to improve our health care system? Some of the roles we can play to improve our health care include:

- Vaccinate our children, elderly, and the immune-compromised relatives
- Practice good hand washing procedures because it is reported to be the most efficient way to avoid infection.
- Practice a healthy lifestyle free of alcohol and smoking.
- Drink enough water to avoid dehydration related diseases.
- Exercise to keep our mind and body in healthy condition.

- Eat healthy foods riched in fruits, nuts, and vegetables while avoiding animal fat and refined sugars that increase our weight index and diseases factors.
- Follow healthy dental hygiene.
- Visit a clinician as often as needed.
- Talk to our doctors about potential lifestyles, genetic predisposition, and change of treatment regimen that can improve health.
- Trust that doctors are not out there to there to hurt us, but they are the best people to trust when it comes to our health.
- Pressure lawmakers to provide administrative standards that promote good health.
- Encourage our religious leaders to invite clinicians to educate community members about health care issues.
- Trust that God's love has given us our doctors, religious leaders, and political leaders to help us live a healthy and comfortable even during our transition to death.

If we combine the above with our own personal battle for a healthy lifestyle, each person that compose American household will be happy. Since happiness is the purpose of life, family will be a fun place, and we will continue to enjoy living on this blessed land of opportunity. When there is joy in families, communities are on fire for progress. When all communities combine their pursuit of happiness with each other, harmony will be restored in America who used to care about each of her children.

Other Reasons Why Private and Public Health Plan Options Can and Should Co-Exist

- If Fox News and MSNBC can co-exist, private and public health plan options can and should co-exist.
- If Ivy League and public university can co-exist, private and public health plan options can and should co-exist.
- If public/VA and private hospitals can co-exist, private and public health plan options can and should co-exist.
- If University of Miami and Jackson Memorial Hospital can co-exist, private and public health plan options can and should co-exist.
- If Medicare/Medicaid and BlueCross & Shield can co-exist, private and public health plan options can and should co-exist.
- If Shaquille O'Neil and Kobe Bryant can co-exist, private and public health plan options can and should co-exist.
- If Michelle Obama and Hillary can co-exist, private and public health plan options can and should co-exist.
- If Dick Cheney and Collin Powell can co-exist, private and public health plan options can and should co-exist.

- If Michigan and Texas NAFTA can co-exist, private and public health plan options can and should co-exist.
- If Sarah Palin and Chris Matthew can co-exist, private and public health plan options can and should co-exist.
- If Keith Olbermann and Rush Limbaugh can co-exist, private and public health plan option can and should co-exist.
- If Professor Gates and Officer Cowley can co-exist, private and public health plan options can and should co-exist.
- If Democrats and Republicans can co-exist, private and public health plan options can and should co-exist.
- If a French President can become pro-American, private and public health plan option can and should co-exist.
- If Alcoholics and Adventists can co-exist, private and public health plan options can and should co-exist.
- If NYC Taxi and Subway can co-exist, private and public health plan options can and should co-exist.
- If Holland Tunnel and G.W. Bridge can co-exist, private and public health plan options can and should co-exist.
- If Adventist and the alcoholic pork eaters of Iowa can co-exist, private and public health plan option can and should co-exist.
- If Amtrak and Grey Hound can co-exist, private and public health plan options can and should co-exist.
- If Mac and PC can co-exist, private and health plan options can and should co-exist.
- If Chicago Shied Aquarium and Chattanooga Aquarium co-exist, private and public health plan options can and should co-exist.
- If University of Iowa and Florida Memorial University co-exist, private and public health plan options can and should co-exist.
- If conservative Americans and Mexicans can co-exist, private and public health plan options can and should co-exist.
- If Sabbath keepers and Sunday keepers can co-exist, private and public health plan options can and should co-exist.
- If wind and solar energy can co-exist, private and public health plan options can and should co-exist.
- If doctors and lawyers can co-exist, private and public health plan options can and should co-exist.
- If December 24th sale and January 24th bill can co-exist, private and public health plan options can and should co-exist.
- If the US Soccer team can be the 2009 Confederation Cup finalist, anything is possible when we have a school girl representing US diplomacy. That is why health care reform with both private and public options is possible.

Chapter 5

THEY ARE JUST NOT THAT INTO
HEALTH CARE REFORM

If you are not changing, you are dying because there is no stationary phase in life. If a bell out for the greedy Wall Street executives, the careless Banks, and the outdated car industry needed a bell out that was imminent, Health care reform is more imminent than those industry. Although bell out was not part of the vote for change, the American people compromised to help the big guys and wait for their turn. Now is the turn of the American people to get a health care bell out. We have no time to wait any longer for a change we have voted for. We voted for health care, immigration, and education reform. We need result now because delay is the biggest enemy of progress. If we wait any longer, extremists will kill the health care bill like they did with President Clinton and take over congress and senate for another 10 years. Instead of worrying about their re-election in 2011, lawmakers should do what they were elected for: helping the White House to bring change in Washington. If congress fails to act, the American people will lose interest in election again like it was in 2002. If Obama does not reform health care, immigration, and education, he should not even think of the American supports that when against the gradient and the odds to make the Iowa vote happen. Washington lawmakers need to know that only the people can elect, even if all lobbyists are behind them.

As this debate is going on, America can sense that change is hard to happen. That is why, we voted for the Hollywood-like charismatic leader to call upon lawmakers to act, instead of talk. We have had enough talk; we need action. If congress can go on a 30-day-recess while Americans cancel their vacation to make ends meet and struggle to pay past due health care bill, we can all see that they are not yet ready for change. Until we elect other lawmakers to take over Washington, we need some action on health care now. Do we elect lawmakers to work their way toward re-election or to help us reaching the American dream? Maybe, It's time to have a more attractive Hollywood-like House Speaker and Senate Majority Leader, so what happen in Vegas won't be heard in D.C.

How About the Republicans, Are they Into Health Care Reform?

Republicans are just not that into health care reform. Why then? Senator Kennedy spent 50 years in writing hundreds of health care reform versions that the Michael Steel corporation has managed to destroy. Democrats have agreed over 120 amendments on this last health reform bill written by the Senator before he died, in order to find an agreements with the party of no. We all know that they are actually planning on strategies for attacking my writings, because I have chosen to be on the moderate side, instead of the of Michael Steel, and Rush Limbaugh. Wouldn't it better for them to sit down with Dr. S. Gupta, Dr. Nancy, and Dr. Howard Dean, in order to better understand the health care bill before planning to add another 240 amendments to this last piece of health care art that produced political stress on the neurons of Senator Kennedy, because reform is not in favor of the insurance and drug companies they are lobbying for! Even if Democrats put everything republicans want in the health reform bill, they still won't vote for it because they are not that into health care reform. It is outrageous for Americans to spend $6,000 more in health care than any industrialized country on earth, while ranking #30 on medical care, and to hear the Republicans say that we have affordable health care. As we said earlier, since delay is the enemy of progress, Republicans are only slowing the bill down until the kill it and thus kill the Obama legacy. From the financial, housing, and car industry bell out, we can see that they have becoming a party of NO. Democrats should turn this adversity into advantages and the opportunity to eliminate fear tactics from Washington by passing the health care bill, with or without Republicans, because there is no such thing call payback in politics if Oprah can elect the most attracted president while Michelle still has an exclusive husband.

More Facts Proven that they Are Just not that into Reform.

- The US Senate is only playing political game over health care reform, by the changing the rhythm from public option to co-op to postponing for later.
- Senator Joe Lieberman, who voted against the change Senator Kennedy supported till death, is advocating postponing the health care debate until he stab the democrats again.

- Conservative media is been manipulated by special interest groups to shut down a real debate.
- The health care debate is between the White House and the majority congress, versus a Senate that does not want a debate about reform.
- Senate could have reformed health care if they wanted reform despite opposition because the Democrats have the majority, the White House, the Media, and the American people.
- Rush Limbaugh and Glenn Peck are using the conservative Americans for high rating of their shows and personal gains about health care.
- Democrats need to ignore bipartisan to change America, if they don't want to lose the reform opportunity that is going away in case they lost the majority.
- If Democrats don't pass health care and immigration reform, they will lose power for decades, and thus no reform will be possible, like it happened in the past 30 years.
- Using abortion to attack health reform is inaccurate and this is a deceiving fear tactic because the Supreme court has already ruled that abortion should not be funded by federal fund.
- Although illegal immigrants need health care, it is unjust to protest reform because illegal immigrants which could also benefit since illegal immigrants are less than 4% of of the American population.

Chapter 6

IMMIGRATION: A HEALTH CARE, FINANCIAL, AND NATIONAL SECURITY ISSUE

Although Michael Jackson used of a surgical anesthesia to fall asleep eternally was not typically coming to the US through broken boarder, we can arguable say that H1N1 virus might have sneaked into the American soil through the broken Mexican boarder. If we do not fix the immigration border as soon as possible, we will open doors to illegal infection while the intelligents and the righteous wait for years to be called to the land of opportunity.

Although the American people would be outraged to hear that a health care reform would have possible coverage for illegal Immigrant, as a health care professional, we should get the record straight, despite its controversy. If America is truly looking for good health, it should provide health care for all, no matter their immigration status. There are many reasons for that. First of all, before we can logically say illegal immigrant should have no benefits on health care reform, we would need to look at the American history, constitution, and economy. I am not going to talk about the same old fact that America was built by immigrants or America is a country of immigrants. What country on earth, did not, once upon a time, started by some foreigners who came to establish to that new land? This is the worse non-sense reason to help the illegal immigrant. The real reasons start with the constitution. Our laws say that anyone who is born in America is an American. This also implies to the sons and daughters of the illegal aliens that are working $12/day at the Florida orange or the California apple fields. Are you telling me that their children can get H1N1 flu vaccine this coming Fall, whereas the parents who are living in the same one-bed-efficiency will not be vaccinated? Do you know that the parents are those who will first be exposed to the virus while being exploited by the American pork industry? Do you know that vaccine only protect you about 90% against infection? What about the 10% viral genome that is floating around the bed of child of the illegal parent? Are you going to tell me that we should only hope that the 10% odds does not happen? What if it happen in at least one illegal immigrant household, whose children go to the same magnet school as your smart children? Do you know that signs and symptoms of virus infection only show two weeks after infection, when T-Cell and Macrophages are already playing the overtimes? Do you know that when the first child is diagnosed with H1N1, Influenza, hepatitis, or any other infection, he or she already pasted it to the whole school, neighborhood, and mall he or she visited in the past 15 days?

It is unfortunate that the public health authority has been "playing safe" by not addressing this issue as it should have been. America, we need to make a wake up call to Washington to reform the immigration system, even before health care reform is completed because, no other change is possible in this country unless the gates are controlled, everyone in this land is insured, and all who come to America is evaluated. This president need to have a talk with public health expects before considering postponing the immigration reform, because we will be running our time and money for the economy, health care, and education, if we leave behind the illegal immigrants that count for 4% of the American population. We know this issue is not were Washington scores good political point, but we also know that if we fight for point more than learning, we will never score the good final grade. That is why, immigration reform should not be delayed and this government should be a multi-task administration where two issues could be discuss at the same table, just as we do it at every kitchen table. If we have to postpone immigration reform in order to reform health care, aren't we doing the same thing we blame McCain for doing: canceling his campaign in order to discuss financial crisis. Those in hatred of illegal immigrants who are lying about health reform in saying that it would promote euthanasia, may have a plan to apply euthanasia against illegal immigrant or sterilized all illegal immigrants so that they won't have children in America. Since they are always right on the extreme right, you never know if they will not propose this anti-immigrant plan on the "O'Reilly Factor Show." I am not saying that illegal immigrant should be provided US Citizenship, but I am saying that they should be provided US health standard of living, as long as they are on our soil.

Immigration is also a matter of national security. Although my Yankee stars and Michael Phelps are able to obtain illegal drugs from the illegal alien, this does not give those supporters of our Olympic MVP the right to corrupt our youth and deteriorate our national standards. Until we fix our northern and southern borders, crime and violence will always over-rule our laws, because criminals can murder in America, shut down our plans, and destroy our American value, while they can safely cross the Mexican and Canadian border toward a joyful life. Instead of investing in big Black Water firms to go after the bad guys in the Middle East, we need to start investing in helping the Mexican government to chase those illegal drug cartels. Instead of spending in airport security, we need to spend in border patrol so that the Canadian border, where terrorists cross onto America, can be patrolled. What do we really do for our national security to invest in airport security, whereas the southern wildlife doesn't even have a monkey to control the entry of banana to America, nor does any deer is available when meat is coming from Canada.

Do you really think that American farmers want to fix the broken immigration system? Who is going to take care of their orange and tomato fields at the wage of $15/day? Since corporate farmers don't want to provide adequate pay to American workers, they are happy with the broken immigration system so that they can exploit the illegal aliens with underpaid salary without benefits. It is interesting to see that Jeb and Charlie are very famous in Florida by helping farmers to continue that human right violation that has become a human trafficking issue. In Florida, as long as you can speak Spanish, you can have a $15/day job, and the state government has done all it can to destroy the single immigrant process that works: the e-Verify. E-Verify is a federal internet service that provides employers the possibility to instantly verify the authenticity of a state or federal Identification card. Before e-Verify, people used fake ID and shared ID among family and friends in order to work in America. Although this program has been one of the most efficient immigration procedure, because of its lack of political supports, it has not been supported by private and governmental agencies. Politics has been so much more important than actual American issues, when then Senator Hillary Clinton supported the plan of of great Governor Pitzer to provide driver's license to illegal immigrants, she has to quickly pulled off her support for that proposal, while illegal immigrants are the major cab drivers in New York City. That is, whether we allow them to live the American lifestyle or not, they will live it because they are already here. That is why we need to incorporate them to the society, and make them pay taxes, and disciplinary fee so that they can fully integrate themselves in the American society. Who knows if the next president, US Senator, or Supreme Court Judge will not be the son or daughter of an illegal immigrant? Furthermore, spending billions of dollars in fencing the border is not the solution because concentration gradient is more powerful than artificial standards; that is, even with the best national security standards, if people are dying of poverty in the other sides of the border, they will manage to defy the law of physics to come to the land of opportunity. That is why, we need to help poorer countries so that they can provide for their own people; otherwise, millions will keep trying to swim to our shores, until they can find a breathe of life. The pyramid of Maslow has thought us that we cannot fight against basic physiological needs, especially if their own leader, like former Mexican President, Vicente Fox, who rather published a "survival border crossing manual," instead of providing basic needs to his own people. They best fight would be win in helping others to be self-sufficient, so that their jealousy won't turn against us.

Chapter 7

THE TOP 15 KILLERS OF THE AMERICAN PEOPLE.

The Chart of the Top 15 American Killers

Disease	Signs & Symptoms	# of death each year	Cause & risk factors	Prevention
Heart Diseases	Pain in jaw, neck, or back. Feeling weak, light-headed, or faint. Chest pain or discomfort. Pain or discomfort in arms or shoulder. Shortness of breath.	649,000	Blood cholesterol levels High Blood Pressure Diabetes Mellitus Tobacco use Diet Physical inactivity Obesity Alcohol hereditary	Decrease cholesterol Decrease blood pressure Avoid smoking and smokers Healthy diet Exercise Health weight Stop drinking alcohol

Cancer	Varies with type: Shortness of breath Lost of appetite Lost of weight Lost of libido Weight gain Constipation Infections	559,000	Hereditary Chemical exposure Alcohol Diet Tobacco use Sun UV-Wave	Avoid smoking and smokers Healthy diet Exercise Healthy weight Stop drinking alcohol HPV vaccine Avoid sun exposure
Stoke	Sudden numbness Sudden weakness of the face, arms, or legs. Sudden confusion or trouble speaking or understanding others. Sudden trouble seeing Sudden trouble walking, dizziness, or loss of balance or coordination. Sudden severe headache with no known cause	143,000	High blood pressure Heart diseases Atrial Fibrillation Diabetes Tobacco Use Blood Cholesterol Levels Alcohol Genetic Risk Factors	Prevent and control high blood pressure Prevent and control diabetes Avoid smoking and smokers Treat atrial fibrillation Prevent and control high blood cholesterol No alcohol use Maintain a healthy weight Regular Physical Activity Diet and nutrition Genetic Risk Factors

Respiratory diseases	Shortness of breath Wheezing Tridor Rhonchi Crackles Dullness Hyper-resonance Frematus Ergophony	130,000	Smoking Infection Asbestos Obesity Chemical exposure Alcohol Genetic Risk Factors	Avoid smoking & smokers Vaccination Avoid chemical exposure Healthy weight Avoid alcohol
Accident	N/A	114,000	Motor vehicle Workplace Slippery Cleaning gun	Safe driving Use work safely standards Walk with caution Avoid gun repair at home
Diabetes Mellitus	Frequent urination Excessive thirst Unexplained weight gained or weight loss Extreme hunger vision changes & dry skin Tingling in extremities & frequent infection	74,000	Being obese Genetic predisposition Mostly non-Caucasian Prior history of gestational diabetes High blood pressure High LDL cholesterol Physical inactivity	Healthy weight Lower cholesterol Lower blood pressure Exercise Healthy diet

Alzheimer's disease	Difficulty with new memories. Trouble finding words. Lose spark or zest for life. Lose judgment about money. Shorter attention span and less motivation lose way going to familiar places. Resists change. Trouble organizing and thinking logically. Asks repetitive questions.	71,000	Over 55 year old Genetic predisposition High blood pressure High cholesterol Diabetes	Intellectual activities Lower cholesterol Lower blood pressure Exercise Healthy weight
Influenza and Pneumonia	Fever Headache Productive Coughing Meningitis Shortness of breath Wheezing Weakness Dullness	62,000	Viral infection Bacterial infection HIV/AIDS Immune Disease Contact with infected people Contact with infected materials	Vaccination Hand washing Avoid contact with infected people Use glove to Cary materials

Kidney Diseases	Hematurea Polyurea Polydipsia Uncontrolled blood pressure	43,000	Alcohol Smoking Diabetes Lupus Drug toxicity	Avoid alcohol Avoid smoking and smokers Control diabetes Healthy weight Control drug use
Septicemia	Bacterial infections	34,000	pathogens	hand washing
Suicide	N/A	31,000	Loneliness Stress Anxiety Depression Mental disease	Stress management Social support Anti-depressant Physical activities
Liver disease	Jaundice Upper abdominal pain Large abdomen Weight gain Loss of vision Uncontrolled blood pressure	27,000	Alcohol drinking Smoking Chemical exposure Drug toxicity Food toxicity	Prevent and control high blood pressure Avoid smoking and smokers Prevent and control high blood cholesterol No alcohol use
hypertension	Exercise intolerance Headache Loss of vision	24,000	Smoking Obesity High Cholesterol Alcohol Diabetes	Avoid smoking and smokers Healthy weight Exercise Control cholesterol

Parkinson's disease	Resists change. Trouble organizing and thinking logically. Difficulty with new memories. Lose judgment about money. Shorter attention span and less motivation lose way going to familiar places. Asks repetitive questions. Trouble finding words. Lose spark or zest for life.	19,000	Heredity Over 50 year old	Intellectual activities Exercise Healthy lifestyles
homicide	N/A	17,000	Gun use Gangster activities Illicit drugs Alcohol Prostitution	Control gun use Avoid alcohol Avoid illicit drugs Avoid woman trafficking

In looking at the above most common diseases and their related annual death in America, we can deduce that alcohol and drugs are the two single most dangerous products in the American society. Having said that, we can arguably deduce that the following are the #1 Enemies of America's Health

- Smoking: is one of the primary cause of the most common health issues in America.
- Alcohol: alcohol does not only affect the physical health, it is also affecting our thinking.
- Fast food: is the major cause of obesity and the complication of health risks in America.
- Prescription and illicit drugs: has not only killed our minds, it has destroyed our city.

- Lack of health education: education could help many sexually transmitted diseases.
- Pornography: pornography has destroyed the sexual health in American family. Unfortunately, long before a mom teaches her son about sexual life, pornography has already taken away their sexual behaviors at the first few years of life, when the mind and characters are being built. TV, internet, and the "Play Boy" are the biggest enemies of the youth before adolescent age. This is why academic performance and moral behavior are proven to be reversely proportional in the life of children who have more access to the entertainment industry.
- Divorce: has become so common that America don't realize it is a mental death penalty and an homicidal action to spouse and children. Just like heart disease, obesity, abortion, and homosexuality have been slowly killing our, heart, body, mind, and economy, divorce has slowly becoming an American epidemic.

The Most destructive social diseases in America:

- Money: love of money have taking priority over family and moral values.
- Power: people do anything to be in charge, even when the society suffers.
- Stress: is the primary cause of disease complication and immunity deactivator.
- Religious nuts: spiritual fruits of love are not present among religious nuts in the society.
- War: attacks to foreign country have destroyed young soldiers and the American values.
- Abortion: killing embryos and fetus has become an American's way of genocides.
- Politics: leaders, on their power greed, care more about re-election than administration.
- Laziness: welfare should have been a seasonal support but has become a lifestyles.
- Homosexuality: When kids go to college, they come back with homosexual anti-biological degree
- Too much food: Americans eat 3 times the amount of food people eat in other countries.
- Prescription drugs: more people die on drug than any disease in American health care.
- Extramarital sex: married governors and unmarried youth have sex to whoever.

- Domestic violence: suicide and homicide has become the pathway of family violence.
- The jail & prison system: Terrorists obtain forgiveness while Americans are never forgiven. Felony people go to prison to learn how to become serial killers.
- The Nursing home system: more elderly get sick and die in nursing home than anywhere

Chapter 8

THE BEST INVESTMENTS

Family & friends

The best short scale and long term investment is investing in human being, such as family and friends. Although it is not obvious to see, when we invest in family in friends, we might be making the best investment of our lives. I am not only talking about the little Johnny that we bail out from juvenile jail for felony, but I am also talking about helping Johnny's mom with our financial and moral supports to better raise the little Johnny. Even when other family members are not living to our standards, this does not prevent us from doing whatever we can to help others in the family to reach there goal. From my own experience, I can tell you that I would not be writing this book today, if I didn't obtain the supports of my family and friends. In looking further forward, we can see the power of educating our young people by looking at the profile of our current president. Despite his youth life was filled with sorrows and challenges, when his mother pasted away, his grand parents could have had any stereotypic excuses not to support him. As we all can arguably admit, he has become the icon for American prestige around the world, even with his challenged youth.

No matter how rough can a family be, a violent father, a weak mother, and rebellious children may have better purpose of life at home than living in a parentless foster care and shelter. We can arguably say that mothers are better than the best nurses of the hospitals and fathers are the best social workers ever existed. Instead of investing in social care, adoption, and juvenile services, we need to promote family bonding by helping fathers, mothers, and children to communicate and interact on each other's needs and goals. Instead of taking the baby away from mentally and behaviorally challenged parents, we should help those parent to become better parents. We are not advocating anti-adoption. As the matter of fact, all children deserve a home; if their parent die, it is our moral and spiritual responsibility to take this child to our home. On the other hand, children who have parent should grow up with their parents. If we want to help those children, instead of try to take them away from the reality of their lives, we would better help them by helping their parent with a fresh start or re-start. This start might be in the helping of providing food, finding a job, building a home, or paying for academic expenses. What does it help with to take the smartest child away from the parents to live with a stranger who is rich and successful while siblings and parents are being destroyed by misery and violence? Do you think that this child that is swimming in wealth and comfort, would ever be happy while their love ones are dying? Genetic bonding is the most powerful bond that is ever existed. Parental connection is the greatest network of all technology. That is why America will be healthier and even stronger, when family values are the priority of our daily living.

Community Investment

Another good investment is to belong to a community. What I mean by belonging to a community is to invest on it. Investment is not only about sending a check to the local library or dropping some clothes at the community shelter. Time is the most important property we have. Love requires that we share our most valuable properties to other. It is, sometimes, more powerful and influential to take the HIV test at the local community health center than sending a few grand to finance the project. We don't have to be NBA starts to show that we care for the community; by being the soccer mom or the football dad to those whose father have given up in them and on life, we can make lifelong differences. If we don't obtain the quick reward of getting the House Representative for the next election, we can be sure that our names are in the biggest electoral bullet in heaven.

It is never to early or too late to be involved in community services. Since I was an adolescent, I have been involved in community activities with my father who is still servicing the community where he lives, even today as he is over 73 years of age. When we involve in community outreach, we decrease the crime and violence level in the neighborhood. Community service that promote family values cannot only decrease divorce rate, but it can also prevent many negative consequences of divorce, separation, and domestic violence. Instead of reading books written by heroes who are able to survive family violence and become successful individuals, we can participate in increasing the number of successful individuals who live in rough families and neighborhoods.

Education

From the Illinois Public School System to the scholarship to Princeton, we have the finest First Lady in American history through the power of education. With the failure of the banking, car industry, and the housing market systems, we can arguably admit that education is the most valuable and the most powerful investment. Instead of encouraging our kids and friends to start working at early age, we need to reverse that pattern by encouraging young people to go to college and pursue a professional degree. When it comes to High School, it is unacceptable to let youth people giving up on America by dropping out of school. It is sad to know that a third of American minority children have dropped out of High School. This drop out rate is not only increasing the prison rate, but also the drawback of the American economy. That is why, the government and the private industry need to spend more in education, starting from kindergarten through doctorate so that America can reclaim the leadership role in education around the world. That is also why, we need reform in our education system when student grant fund can be more efficient and student loans can be more affordable. It is unacceptable to have a student graduate from college with 100,000 dollars of debt on a market where high paying job for students are disappearing. Education reform should be the next priority of the actual government because no other reform will be sufficient and efficacious if education is not the basis of its foundation.

For those who are planning to go to college of graduate school, here is a few advises that might be helpful along the way:

If you are still in high school, start taking college Summer programs to help you understand the opportunity in each field. While the medical and the electronic fields are the most needed fields in the society, when the economy is back on track, the financial world might become an influential field.

GPA is still considered as the most important factor that determine a college or graduate school admission. Instead of focusing on the extracurricular activities that we have told to consider, we need to make sure we have the 3.5 or above GPA that is required by most institutions across the board.

If you are looking at the medical option, it is best to start looking at your school selection during you sophomore year in High School for the best pre-medical program. During the second semester of your sophomore college year, you need so look at MCAT, PMAT, LSAT, and GRE programs that might fit you need and finance the most. By the 1st semester of you junior college year, you should be able to have all admission applications submitted, so that you can be on the early bird admission list.

Student visa is another way the government can both improve immigration and education in America. Student visa off-spring has provided to America the first American president that is is imported from Africa instead of China. If we provide more student visa, we can attract the richest and the brightest to our educational system. Since the foundation of our great land, America has had the democracy, the financial security, and human right policies to attract all people to our shores. Helping young people by granting them student visa and/or scholarship, will give every intelligent young person around the world, the same opportunity the Cubans have, even when they illegally cross our Southeastern borders. Like Senator Martinez and President Obama prove it, if we give others the access to the land of opportunity, the final outcomes will be for our benefits. This is the power of love and help, that whoever waters someone will eventually be watered. That is why we should spray the water of our great education throughout the world.

Real Estate Investment

If you wonder where to invest your money during this financial crisis? If you wonder when to buy your first or tenth house, now is the time to invest in real estate. Real estate has become one of the greatest areas of opportunity. Because of the high foreclosure rate and the credit crisis, builders and homeowners are giving out bargains. Now is the time to buy a house under 70% of its value. If you are buying you first house, you can look for that 10% credit that the government is giving out. I know you don't trust the government enough to take money for clunkers, house, energy, and Wall Street. The sad thing is that, we all are going to pay for it whether we take it or not. That is why, it is best to take that 10% credit from the government before the bill expires in November, instead of paying for the next big guy, who get it all from Washington.

If you want to invest, it is best to buy another house that can give you a 20% equity within 2 years, adding to the rental fee you collect instead of investing in the stock market that will take 20% of your fund in potential market crash. If you wonder whether Trump still believe that real estate is the way to go, buy a property for 10 grand and rent it for one grand/month, you will see what is your profit in the 11th month.

Working in the real estate and mortgage industry during my undergraduate college years thought me about the powerful housing business. You don't even have to think like a billionaire to make billions in the housing industry. All you need to do is to start low, built fast, and invest smart, at the most targeted locations you want to buy and resell. If you want to rent your property, it is best to go in smaller towns where your mortgage will not even reach ¼ of you profits on rental. Townhouse and duplex are the most powerful money making in the rental system. Even the smallest investment can, with times, build so much wealth that you will not need the 9 to 5 or the overnight to reach the American dreams and become successful.

Mutual Fund, RIA, and Stock Market

Unlike the beliefs of the past few decades, the usual Mutual Fund, RIA, and Stock Market should only be investment made with fund that is not needed within 10 years. If you have been saving for little Johnny to go to college while he is still in elementary school, it is wise to invest in this flexible market. However, if you are looking for quick profits, you should look at other options where benefits would be larger at the time you need it. Another stressful drawback is the stock market investments are too unstable. On this kind of investment, each hour we look at the ups and downs of the market opening and closing, we wonder whether our money is safe enough. Such stressful financial life is not good for our mental and physical health. With the US News on new scams on the Wall Street, the investment market have not yet created the confidence we need, in order to invest our fund in the market for short term profits.

Chapter 9

THINGS WE THOUGHT YOU SHOULD KNOW

Why Hillary Clinton Believes she Will Never Win the Presidency?

- She is the symbol of old politics
- She is called school girl by foreign leaders
- She was trying to act like the average blue color Americans while she symbolized the New American Elites.
- She stood in the way of Rev. J. Wright by pretending that she knew and felt what the black people have gone through, while she never got a white Friend or teacher who got profiled or stopped for having a house, a driver's license, or a doctorate.
- During the presidential campaign, unlike Sarah Palin, she unsuccessfully tried to pimp out her daughter Chelsea to buy the Hollywood stars.
- She does not know what it feels to be black whereas all people in the Mall would watch over their wallet when a black person is around.
- She wanted to be black without knowing that Hollywood only has black character as the local gangster.

Why John McCain Mainly Lost the Election?

- He could not do two things at once by cancelling his election campaign in order to pursuit a dialogue about the financial crisis.

- He was told to believe that the fundamentals of our economy is strong while President Clinton and President Bush sent our economic fundamentals to China through NAFTA.
- He choose Sarah Palin to help with D.C. While Palin didn't even know Washington Bully Politics.
- Palin was attacking the Media who have been selecting presidents for America for the past few decades.
- John McCain believes only the extremist Muslims we used to sponsor against Russia and Iran are evil, while crimes in Phoenix made his wife buy an airplane to move around Arizona.
- McCain was the accidental Republican Nominee because Romney's strongest economic strength was not needed until after the Primary election with the financial melt down.
- Republicans let religious extremists control the policy of the party.
- Republicans promote fair and anger that would create physiological changes that facilitate fighting and fleeing among the American people.
- Mike Huckabee failed to carry the primary on the economy and health care reform by talking about foreign wars that are the strength of McCain.
- The previous administration has used torture and mental abuse to interrogate prisoners, without knowing that abused individuals would say and do anything to avoid further torture.
- McCain has trade his title of best Capitol Hill politician with Senator Linsey Graham for a VP nominee who didn't know the destructive power of Washington D.C.

Who Said What!

- Who said Linsey Graham is not the best Southern Republican for bipartisan?
- Who said anyone on the bench is better qualified than Sonia Sotomayor?
- Who said Howard Dean is not the best M.D. the democratic party needed to get back to American hearts.
- Who said that Michelle Obama is not the smartest American First Lady?
- Who said that Lucia Whalen should not be part of the White House Inter-racial Beer Summer of Racial Profile because she started it with the 911 call on Professor Gates?
- Who said experience is the only key to success while Dick Cheney is the most experience and the worse recorded Vice-President?
- Who said that President Obama is a black president while his mother is white?

- Who said that the arrested journalists in North Korea and tourists in Iran were not spying on those countries. Unless they are retarded and never watch CNN, and are out of touch not to know that Iran & N Korea are not Canadian borders, unless they are trying to help Bush adding more on Obama's change plan. Although it helped Bill to prove they power of diplomacy even around enemies.
- If a clown like Al Franklen can be elected as US Senator, an ignorant like Rush Limbaugh can one day become the US President.

Fact & truth vs. Myth & Fiction

- 8 cups of water a day is good enough for all : myth
- Prescription drug is the #1 preventable death in America: True
- Government tracks CARS.gov log in on the "Cash for Clunkers" programs: myth
- Euthanasia is the government goals in reforming health care: myth
- Sarah Palin resign to avoid expensive lawsuit spending for the state of Alaska: myth
- John McCain maverick political power ends with the vote against Sonia Sotomayor, health care reform, and stimulus economy: True
- Rush Limbaugh is only destroying our conservative values by attacking his opponents to increase his entertainment rating: true
- Meat diet promote aggressive behaviors: true
- Staring at cute or ugly people would make your unborn beautiful: False
- Rick Sanchez has volunteered to go spying on Cuba and Venezuela during his next vacation: False

We Thought you Should Know:

- CPR should never be done on soft compartments, such as bed and sofa, unless you are Michael Jackson's Dr.
- Do not swim after eating because blood moves away from our muscles toward out Abdomen for digestion, and prevent muscle released after contraction that would drown us.
- Do not let babies in car with closed windows because baby temperature rises very quick till die of hyperthermia.
- Herbal remedies are not FDA approved or tested.
- Alcohol and drugs decrease vision and critical thinking abilities.
- America spends 40% of its health care budget in preventable cardiovascular and heart disease treatment.
- President Obama is not black because his mother was white, he was raised on a white family, and educated around the white scholars; If genetics,

nurturing, education, and lifestyles, are all combined in determining the personality of a person, we can deduce that the president only bought a black skin and walk style from Kenya whereas everyone else buy their stuff in China.

- Michael Jackson's Doctor used Propofol, a surgical anesthetic drug, to put Michael to sleep in initiating black and elderly euthanasia proclaimed by the right wing extremists.
- The American Prison system has failed us and only raised crime and suicidal level in America while California is being bankrupted by spending our tax money to take care of those who murder our family and friends.
- Unlike hospitals and hospices that are respectively saving lives and creating good transition to death, the nursing home system has failed us by mentally and physical killing our elderly and disabled Americans.
- Prison, that is a physical isolation of our criminals, and nursing home, that is a mental isolation of our annoying elderly, are the major locations where infection and disease spread the most in America.
- An American America spends $6,000/year more in health care than any industrialized country around the globe.
- VA health care and US Military Academic, which are federally run health care and academic system, are respectively the best and the finest health care and academic institutions in America.
- If the arrested journalists in North Korea & tourists in Iran were not spying for our government, they most be retarded, and out of touch not to know Iran and N Korea are not Canadian borders, unless they are trying to help bush adding more on Obama's change plan. Although it would help Bill to prove they power of diplomacy even around enemies, we should discourage Rick Sanchez and George Lopez to volunteer to go to Cuba and Venezuela at the expense of Secretary Clinton.
- We need to change the military laws so that the professed openly gays can join the military while receive mental treatments, so that politicians can safely cheat on their wives without any divorce threats or lost of political power. This is because Being gay is a chosen lifestyle or profession just like Cheney's daughter can declare that she is an open lesbian and still able to defy biology to carry a baby.

What if:

- What if you our insurance card was as flexible as your ATM debit card?
- What if your medical record was as flexible as your FICO credit score?
- What if every medical clinic was as flexible as Mc Donald?

- What if your exercise was as constant as your TV time?
- What if your conception made you feel as good as your erection?
- What if the disabled were honored as the Olympic MVP?
- What if Michael Vick's mistake was treated as Michael Phelps's?
- What if politicians had only one term?
- What if lawmakers would serve America ad hard as our troops?
- What if the right wing would administer the Media?
- What if the left wing would obey to God's voice of love?
- What if Israel would stop believe they are the only sovereign country on Earth?
- What if china would have a real worker compensation?
- What if Christians would promote peace instead of appeasing the bullies?
- What if poorest countries and people would obtain interest-free loan from the World bank?
- What if Extremist Muslims would stop the hatred against the West?
- What is knowledge and wisdom would be the reason for power?
- What if everyone would have access to the Cleveland Clinics?
- What if medication would have no side effects?
- What if medical care was available to all people like water and oxygen?
- What if fast foods were fat, cholesterol, and refined sugar free?
- What if science was the major subject on BET, MTV, and all barber shops?
- What if we could vote at the ATM machine?
- What if the democrats did not procrastinate the health care bill until Senator Kennedy passed away?
- What if Caroline Kennedy would agree to become the first female president of America?

I Have a Dream

- I have a dream, When the mind and the soul would be the primary requirement for leadership
- I have a dream, when Iran and America can be friends.
- I have a dream, when gays and lesbians will seek treatment like other mental health patients.
- I have a dream, when North Korea and the West can seat at the same peaceful table for lunch.
- I have a dream, when abortion will no longer be another easy crime out of inconvenient babies.
- I have a dream, when everyone can be insured of basic physiological need and don't have to chase health care, food, and shelter.
- I have a dream, when all immigrants will be legal in America.

- I have a dream, when education will be free for all Americans.
- I have a dream, when all America will stand again as one nation under God.

Being Like the Eagle

Being like the eagle:
Not like the one who does not train the eaglet;
Not like the one who is similar to the pullet;
Not like the one who does not know what is eaglet;
Not like the one whose major task is neglected.

Being like the eagle:
Not like the one whose velocity under its gravity;
Not like the one whose needs are over the community;
Not like the one who is omitting humility;
Not like the one who is deficient in loyalty.

Being like the eagle:
Not like the one who does like to hunt for reptile;
Not like the one does not have a profile;
Not like the one who procrastinates the improved file;
Not like the one who prefer to die than making changes in his lifestyle.

Being like the eagle:
Not like the one who does not want to incise temporary useful wings;
Not like the one who is not decisive in replacing old nails;
Not like the one who is scared of being hurt while changing boots;
Not like the one whose endurance is less valuable than looks.

Being like the eagle:
Not like the one whose pride kills objectives and ambition;
Not like the one whose domicile is too pleasant for shelter conception;
Not like the one who is not standing by for renovation;
Not like the one who is not ready for transformation.

Being like the eagle:
Not like the not one who does not have a dream;
Not like the one who compare nightmare to a dream;
Not like the one who live upon a lie;
Not like the one who does not flirt in the sky;

Being like the eagle:
Not like the one who does not reflect the future;
Not like the one who does not have power;
Not like the one who can not use his power;
Not like the one who does not renew his power.

Being like the eagle:
Being like the eagle who is the pioneer;
Being like the eagle who is the creator;
Being like the eagle who is the rebuilder;
Being like the eagle who is the finisher;

Catherine Flont

You were helping neighbors,
We blamed you as useless;
You fought for our freedom,
We blamed you for your hurt;
You were murdered for us,
We described you as pedant.

You fought for equality,
We pursue inequality;
You are still living like slaves,
We celebrate your liberty;
You burned out for us,
We entitle you: "cancerous."

You sacrificed your life for us,
We declare: it is not worthy!
You destroyed schools for us,
We christen your mediocrity;
You invented hospitality,
We believe you disgust charity.

You prepare priests for us,
We say you are blasphemous;
You sold your revenue for us,
We left you in poor blindness;
You helped us to progress,
We say you destroyed the endocrine.

You symbolized our unity,
We embryolized your diversity;
You were celebrating victory,
We shouted: it is not worthy!
You were worshiping the Majesty,
We assumed you are daughter of iniquity.

You have gotten the medal,
We have taken the reward;
You worked hard as John the Apostle,
We qualify you as Queen Jezebel;
You have the Lord in your side,
We still try to put you aside.

You worked, for many, in the thrones,
We make you sitting upon the bones;
You represented the beautiful ones,
We put you among the ugliest ones;
You are enlightening for success,
We are shouting: for you, no progress!

Dissimilitude

He was born on earth,
Bu He is the creator of the universe;
He was raised in a religious family,
But he is the precursor of faithfulness;
He was asking question,
But he is the answer of every problem;
He was baptized,
But he is the origin of baptism.

He was praying,
But he is the Lord who forgives;
He was tempted,
But he dwells over temptation;
He was worshiping in fellowship,
But he is the glorified Majesty;
He started his ministry while hungry,
But he is the living bread.

He achieved his ministry with thirst,
But he is the inalterable spring of water;
He paid tribute to others,
But he is the king of the world;
He was accused of possessing demon,
But he cursed out a legion;
He was crying,
But he dried out people's tears.

He was accused of violating one Sabbath,
But he is the Master of the Sabbath;
He was carried like a lamb,
But he is the "good shepherd;"
He was crucified,
But his crucifixion introduces a new kingdom;
He was held in a cross,
But his cross symbolizes the everlasting life.

He was abandoned,
But his abandonment saves humanity;
He was crying,
But his tears carry the kingdom of joy;
He was forsaken,
But he is the Omni-Present;
He was killed,
But his death gives life to whoever believed.

He was pierced with a sword
But his mark gives faith to others;
He was buried in a grave,
But he resurrected people from death;
He was watched over by soldiers,
But he gives victory to armies;
He was resurrected,
But his resurrection starts a new beginning.

He was walking with others,
But he is the road to heaven;
He was tired,
But he gives rest to whoever believes;
He was breaking bread,

But is the leaving bread;
He was drinking wine,
But he is the grapefruit of life.

He was caught up to heaven,
But he has the power over gravity;
He ministers in the heaven,
But he is the architect of the heavenly sanctuary;
He is advocating before the father,
But his is the judge and savior of the world;
He went up alone
But he is coming back with the heavenly army.

He is in heaven,
But he hears our sorrow;
He left us in mourning,
But he will destroy grieving;
He left us with an imperfect character,
But he will give us an incorruptible mind;
He left us with a deadly body,
He will dress us with the immortal clothes

The Chicken and the Eagle

Once upon a time, someone found an eagle egg and brought it under a chicken for embryological reproduction. This eagle egg was the fourth to be hatched among nine other chicken eggs; he grew up in the poultry with all the chicks; so that, he never knew he is an eagle. He ate anything that chicks eat, drank anything chicks drink, and slept anywhere with every chick. Hence, he was just like a chick. He did not know what was supposed to be his lifestyle!

One day, he discovered that he was an eagle as soon as another eagle was flying around the poultry in teaching the eaglets how to fly in the sky. He looked at himself in a mirror and found that he was typical to the other eagles; he said:

"Wait a minute! I think I look just like these birds! I think I can do everything they do! If I could believe that I would, I should start!"

He said to an eaglet that admires his good fatty muscle:

"How can your parents teach me how to do these?"

The eaglet looks at him and laughs. The good looking eagle replies:

-"I am not kidding girl; I want to do these!"

"Are you joking fat boy?" Replies the little female eaglet. "Do you mean that at your age, you still cannot do these easy things? As a matter of fact, my parent would love to help you so that you can take care of them when they are retired!"

"Retired? What does an eagle would have to do with retirement plan?" he replied.

"Yes, thicky boy, she says . . . ! Here is the deal buddy! If I let my parent train you, every big fish or reptile you catch, you got to bring them to the family."

-"Fish and reptiles? What do you mean?" He says.

"Nothing . . . are you from a planet different from ours or what?" she asks. Thus, the terrestrial eagle tries to carefully follow the instruction in order to make his first trip to the sky. Every time he moves, there is a chain of fat that brings him back to the planet he belongs to. He could not imagine how come some old eagles have more strength than he does. He starts thinking and no longer has his appetite. All the chickens that admire him for his differentiation among them try to understand and share the sorrow with him; however, this sympathy makes him sadder because no other could understand what he is going through. A rooster approaches him and says:

"Buddy, why don't you accept things how they comes and eat you great corn and mango juice, and have fun while waiting for you day to go to the kitchen pat?"

"Accept, he says! Is there any reason for that. What food or juice would do for me if I lost my body and soul?"

With everyone being sad after his opinion, a chicken says among them:

"A kind word can warm a winter season! Let us talk to him and help him planning for his dreams! May be he could become our redeemer."

"Listen buddy! As I eat and drink, as I am nod off to take a stand. Therefore, if you want to move on, you would rather start looking after your lifestyles and dream . . ." one rooster says.

Feeling supported by his surrounding, the eagle decided that one year from today should be a moment he will fly by. After several trials, he finally gets to fly and observe the beautiful world around him. When he becomes the strongest eagle in the kingdom, he was struggling against his pride to keep his commitment, which requires him to bring food in the household, building new home for the elderly, and request help from others. It is sweet to profess a belief but the action is bitter.

References

National Institutes of Health Web Site
www.nih.gov

The White House Web Site
www.whitehouse.gov
Center for Disease Control Web Site
www.cdc.gov

Google Web Site
www.google.com

Answers.com Online Dictionary
www.answers.com

To Contact the Author or Manager, Send your Messages to:

Charlyhealthreport.com
1828 Foust Street
Chattanooga, TN 37407
Phone: 347-410-5040
Web: *www.Charlyhealthreport.com*
Email: ppcharly@charlyhealthreport.com

www.ingramcontent.com/pod-product-compliance
Lightning Source LLC
Chambersburg PA
CBHW031305280526
45784CB00004B/1997